WORKBOOK FOR APHASIA

Also by Susan Howell Brubaker

Sourcebook for Speech, Language and Cognition
Stimulus Materials for Rehabilitation
Books 1, 2, and 3

Workbook for Cognitive Skills
Exercises for Thought Processing and Word Retrieval

Workbook for Language Skills
Exercises for Written and Verbal Expression

Workbook for Reasoning Skills
Exercises for Cognitive Facilitation

Basic Level Workbook for Aphasia

WORKBOOK FOR APHASIA

EXERCISES FOR THE REDEVELOPMENT OF HIGHER LEVEL LANGUAGE FUNCTIONING

REVISED EDITION

SUSAN HOWELL BRUBAKER, M.S., CCC-SP
Speech and Language Pathology
William Beaumont Hospital
Royal Oak, Michigan

Foreword by MICHAEL I. ROLNICK

Wayne State University Press Detroit

00 99 98 97 96 11 10 9 8 7

Library of Congress Cataloging-in-Publication Data

Brubaker, Susan Howell, date
Workbook for aphasia.

1. Aphasia—Examinations, questions, etc.
2. Aphasics—Rehabilitation—Examinations, questions, etc. I. Title
RC425.B78 1985 616.85'5206 85-91276
ISBN 0-8143-1803-7

CONTENTS

FOREWORD TO REVISED EDITION

This edition incorporates comments and suggestions from speech and language pathologists and educators committed to quality treatment materials.

The most obvious change is in format. A plastic comb binding now allows the manual to open flat, for easier use by patients with motor problems. Within its new cover clinicians will find among the treatment activities three hundred additional stimulus items and over a hundred revisions. Errors have been corrected and instructions to the user clarified. Blank pages have been removed wherever possible to keep the workbook a convenient size. In response to requests, this edition also includes an answer key to exercises which are especially time consuming to check.

Of particular interest to us has been the growing use of this workbook by other health care and educational specialists. Occupational therapists have found it helpful in hospital and educational settings. It has found its way into many bibliographies of rehabilitation literature. Neuropsychologists have utilized it in working with patients with varying forms of brain dysfunction. Numerous reports from teachers of English as a second language indicate that the workbook helps many new Americans communicate better. Learning disorder professionals and special education teachers say that children with dyslexia and other learning problems have been greatly aided by the workbook activities. Even teachers in regular classrooms have reported much success with their students when using this workbook as a tool.

Despite the interest among these diverse audiences, however, the majority of users continue to be speech and language pathologists throughout the country who have made *Workbook for Aphasia* an integral part of their aphasia rehabilitation and cognitive retraining programs. It supplements treatment of patients with higher level language and cognitive dysfunctions. Patients with various forms of neurological disorders have found it most useful during the road to rehabilitation, providing a variety of treatment activities in the clinic and at home. In short, a most useful treatment tool in the rehabilitation of language-impaired adults and children has now been made even more comprehensive and easier to use than ever.

Michael I. Rolnick, Ph.D., Director
Speech and Language Pathology Department
William Beaumont Hospital
Royal Oak, Michigan
July, 1985

FOREWORD

For the aphasic patient, his family, and the consulting speech and language pathologist, an organized and well-rounded rehabilitation program is a primary concern. A number of rehabilitation techniques have been established, over the years, to help the language-impaired individual recover his communicative abilities, and a variety of materials have been published as aids to the clinician. Most of the materials now available are designed principally for the severely aphasic or apraxic individual, whose basic speech and language abilities are quite limited. Materials are also available for the patient who has recovered a certain degree of communicative function, and who needs more advanced stimulation. For the individual with higher level language loss, however, there is a paucity of material. This patient, having relatively little difficulty with reading, writing, oral expression, and general comprehension, requires a balanced, more sophisticated program of language stimulation if he is further to improve his language abilities.

This collection of such higher level language materials was designed as an aid to the speech and language pathologist in his treatment regimen. He will note that while a number of the exercises can be adapted, with slight modifications, for the lower level patient, the manual is tailored to the needs of the patient who has made a significant recovery of his language functions. An experienced clinician may also find that the range of exercises in the manual suggests to him yet other treatment avenues to explore with his patients, as much of the material is flexible enough to be used in more than one way. Many of the exercises ask for responses that may open discussions between the patient and the clinician, thus further enriching the patient's language use. Finally, assignments can be carried out with a minimum of instruction from the clinician, each exercise giving written directions, as well as examples, specifically designed for the patient with higher level language dysfunction.

The speech and language pathologist will find this manual a useful tool in the rehabilitation of the aphasic patient.

Michael I. Rolnick, Ph.D., Director
Speech and Language Pathology Department
William Beaumont Hospital
Royal Oak, Michigan
August, 1978

INTRODUCTION

There has been an ever increasing need for a workbook designed for aphasic patients with higher level reading and writing capabilities. My own clinical experience has been that the patient who has partially lost his language abilities needs much stimulation in reasoning, writing, memory, word recall, and following directions. As each patient may have needs considerably different from the needs of another, the number and kind of materials required by the clinician may be correspondingly great. The speech and language pathologist who is called upon to develop these exercises finds that, while they are desirable as adjuncts to formal treatment sessions and beneficial as concurrent home programs, their actual creation is extremely time-consuming. This manual was written to help fill this need for creative, interesting higher level material.

The manual was designed to be an adaptable clinical tool: the exercises may be used either in treatment sessions or as home assignments, either orally or written, and in individual or group sessions. It presents a selection of diverse materials for a range of specific problems and several levels of involvement.

For all of the exercises the patient must possess some reading skill, but the skill demanded varies as does the type of answer solicited (matching, copying, or the generation of a word, phrase, or sentence). The list of prerequisites following outlines the proficiency a patient must have developed in order to do each exercise. The exercises are divided, according to common logical groupings, into eight target areas. In each target area, exercises in a particular skill are grouped together; the Contents indicates the number of exercises in each group. Each exercise within a group has different questions and may be assigned independently of the others. Every exercise contains about thirty questions or the approximate work effort.

The amount of time needed to complete a question or exercise will naturally differ from patient to patient, so assignments should be adjusted to the individual's rate and capabilities. The clinician will note that each series of exercises increases in difficulty as it progresses and that there are challenging ones throughout the workbook. There are over one hundred exercises, including those in Supplementary Materials.

The first four target areas concentrate on specific language skills, the last four on general knowledge, reasoning, and thinking processes. The Supplementary Materials section contains fifteen shorter exercises. The clinician may want to expand or modify these exercises for work with individual patients.

I should like to acknowledge the following people, who have been most helpful and encouraging in the preparation of this study: Dr. Michael I. Rolnick, for his contributions to this volume; Bonnye D. Howell, and George H. Howell for their encouragement and suggestions; and my patients, who gave purpose to this effort.

PREREQUISITES FOR EACH EXERCISE

The following list is designed to aid the speech and language pathologist in determining which exercises are appropriate for an individual patient; it notes the reading and writing abilities a patient must possess before attempting a given exercise. Clearly, some of the exercises can be worked through by the patient with limited reading ability and no writing ability, while others require solid reading and writing skills, as well as logical reasoning ability.

The exercises have been grouped below into six categories. This is necessarily a rather rough classification system, as certain exercises overlap categories and others may fit only partially. In each case the exercise has been assigned to the category that seemed most appropriate.

Questions require reading a single word or phrase/ Answers require matching or copying a word	Target Area One:	Synonyms, Exercise 1 Antonyms, Exercise 1 Homonyms, Exercise 1 Vocabulary, Exercises 1, 2, 3 Categorizing, Exercise 1
	Target Area Three:	Scrambled Syllables, Exercises 1, 2, 3 Scrambled Words, Exercises 1, 2, 3 Numerical Sequencing, Exercises 1, 2, 3 Alphabetizing, Exercises 1, 2
	Supplementary Materials:	Exercises 2, 3, 4, 5, 6, 15
Questions require reading a sentence/ Answers require matching or copying a word	Target Area One:	Synonyms, Exercise 2 Antonyms, Exercise 2 Homonyms, Exercise 2
	Target Area Two:	Punctuation Morphemic Usage, Exercise 1
	Target Area Three:	Scrambled Words, Exercise 4 Scrambled Sentences, Exercises 1, 2, 3
	Target Area Four:	Comprehension of Instructions Numerical Reasoning

	Target Area Six:	Yes or No Which One Constant Characteristics, Exercise 1 Ordering of Events
	Target Area Seven:	Analogies, Exercise 1 Proverbs, Exercise 1
Questions require reading a single word or phrase/ Answers require writing a single word	Target Area One:	Synonyms, Exercise 3 Antonyms, Exercise 3 Word Formation, Exercises 1, 2 Categorizing, Exercises 2, 3 Abbreviations
	Target Area Two:	Phrase Completions, Exercises 1, 2, 3, 4
	Target Area Three:	Words within Words Numerical Sequencing, Exercise 4
	Target Area Six:	Commonalties, Exercise 1
	Supplementary Materials:	Exercises 1, 11, 12
Questions require reading a single word or phrase/ Answers require writing more than one word	Target Area One:	Homonyms, Exercises 3, 4 Vocabulary, Exercise 4 Dictionary Usage, Exercise 1
	Target Area Two:	Sentence Construction, Exercises 1, 2, 3 Paragraph Construction
	Target Area Four:	Constant Characteristics, Exercise 2 Commonalities, Exercise 2 Syllogisms
	Supplementary Materials:	Exercise 14
Questions require reading a sentence/ Answers require writing one word	Target Area Two:	Morphemic Usage, Exercises 2, 3 Phrase Completions, Exercise 5
	Target Area Four:	Specific Directions
	Target Area Five:	General Facts, Exercise 1
	Target Area Seven:	Intangibles Analogies, Exercise 2
	Supplementary Materials:	Exercises 7, 8, 9, 10
Questions require reading a sentence/	Target Area One:	Dictionary Usage, Exercise 2
	Target Area Two:	Morphemic Usage, Exercise 4

Answers require writing more than one word	Target Area Four:	Listing Steps
	Target Area Five:	Why Questions What Questions When Questions Where Questions Who Questions How Questions General Facts, Exercise 2
	Target Area Six:	Reasonable Conclusions Similarities and Differences, Exercises 1, 2 Main Differences
	Target Area Seven:	Incongruities Proverbs, Exercises 2, 3
	Target Area Eight:	Completions Descriptions Opinions Hypothetical Situations
	Supplementary Materials:	Exercise 13

Target Area 1
WORD USAGE

One of the most common characteristics of the aphasic patient is a loss of word finding ability commonly called dysnomia. Damage to the cerebral structure which results in word loss is a frustrating condition, causing both the patient and his listener much difficulty.

This target area gives the dysnomic patient specific exercises for word usage and word recall problems. There is a wide range of semantic choice: simple, everyday words are presented in addition to those that are relatively unfamiliar. Several formats are employed, to give interest and challenge to each exercise. Most higher level aphasic patients should be able to work through these exercises with some ease. The final section calls for the patient's use of a dictionary, a helpful tool for the patient who needs an outside source to aid him in performing certain language activities. Several exercises in the Supplementary Materials section may be used in conjunction with this target area.

The majority of exercises in Target Area One can be adapted for oral use, and the difficulty of a given exercise controlled by eliciting true-false or multiple choice responses from the patient. This target area is particularly suited to those individuals who can work with single words but who have trouble with syntax. Eleven of the exercises have multiple choice answers, seven exercises require only a one word answer, and the remaining four ask that a sentence be written for the answer. Because of the number of exercises using the simpler reading, writing, or matching skills, this target area is the one perhaps most easily modified for patients with more severe language disturbances.

M.R.

Target Area 1: Synonyms, Exercise 1

DIRECTIONS: Circle the word below the phrase whose meaning is the closest to the word in dark type.

EXAMPLE: **Huge** means the same as

late (gigantic) tiny

1. **Large** means the same as

   up big elephant

2. **Go** means the same as

   stay leave play

3. **Start** means the same as

   begin engine exit

4. **Lift** means the same as

   up lower raise

5. **Soiled** means the same as

   ashes dirty clean

6. **Allow** means the same as

   permit stop exhibit

7. **Donate** means the same as

   breathe give expect

8. **Repair** means the same as

   relax fix crush

9. **Journey** means the same as

   trip marathon raid

10. **Ship** means the same as

package utensil boat

11. **Tempest** means the same as

storm vehicle nuisance

12. **Sad** means the same as

unhappy moody angry

13. **Finish** means the same as

begin end European

14. **Meet** means the same as

meat enter encounter

15. **Aid** means the same as

accept help give

16. **Yell** means the same as

whisper talk shout

17. **Pretty** means the same as

nervous ugly beautiful

18. **Labor** means the same as

sleep arbor work

19. **Cry** means the same as

laugh weep scatter

20. **Pleasant** means the same as

sad unhappy nice

21. **Afraid** means the same as

scared flat elated

---

22. **Courageous** means the same as

exciting brave loving

---

23. **Detest** means the same as

hate like think

---

24. **Envious** means the same as

tired shy jealous

---

25. **Funny** means the same as

exciting humorous sad

---

26. **Pupil** means the same as

student baby oath

---

27. **Shy** means the same as

healthy bashful smiling

---

28. **Beverage** means the same as

baggage flower drink

---

29. **Adult** means the same as

youngster grownup girl

---

30. **Collide** means the same as

habit listen crash

---

31. **Enormous** means the same as

huge wee furry

32. **Champion** means the same as

loser winner entrant

---

33. **Chef** means the same as

cook chief bartender

---

34. **Pair** means the same as

pare couple trio

---

35. **Tardy** means the same as

tired late early

---

36. **Reliable** means the same as

factual dependable practical

---

37. **Qualified** means the same as

specified drunk competent

---

38. **Shake** means the same as

tremble bake shoulder

---

39. **Coarse** means the same as

smooth course rough

---

40. **Urban** means the same as

city rural suburban

---

41. **Joy** means the same as

sadness happiness bitterness

---

42. **Conceal** means the same as

eat give hide

43. **Rock** means the same as

boulder sand water

---

44. **Antique** means the same as

new ancient moldy

---

45. **Precisely** means the same as

dubiously exactly maybe

---

46. **Apparatus** means the same as

building equipment vegetable

---

47. **Ruin** means the same as

demolish empty fill

---

48. **Gossip** means the same as

rumor question goal

---

49. **Mimic** means the same as

imitate like accept

---

50. **Competent** means the same as

available capable understanding

Target Area 1: Synonyms, Exercise 2

DIRECTIONS: Circle the word below the sentence whose meaning is the closest to the word in dark type.

EXAMPLE: The **huge** elephant was in his cage.

little friendly (big)

1. It was **considerate** of the woman to think of her sick neighbor.

   pleasant thoughtful awful

---

2. I have always **yearned** for a trip to Europe.

   wished asked expected

---

3. Always obey the traffic **laws.**

   lights rules policemen

---

4. We rode in a red **vehicle** to the restaurant.

   car chair carton

---

5. She bought herself some new spring **apparel.**

   buttons flowers clothing

---

6. The new building was **erected** in 11 months.

   built vacated painted

---

7. Before dinner, the children were **grouchy.**

   hungry crabby happy

---

8. The factory **manufactured** plastic bottles.

   made equipped bought

---

9. I bought a new pair of plaid **pants.**

   shoes slacks lamps

10. He was a **graduate** of Michigan State University.

alumnus student professor

---

11. My **luggage** was lost on the plane.

box purse suitcase

---

12. **Dinner** will be served at seven o'clock.

supper snacks lunch

---

13. The **thief** stole some jewelry from the store.

robber salesman baby

---

14. I **remember** when knickers were popular.

see recall wonder

---

15. The little girl was too **timid** to ask for more.

sad tired shy

---

16. **Inexpensive** lobster is hard to find.

nutritional cheap packaged

---

17. It was a very **ugly** dress.

unattractive large colorful

---

18. There was **adequate** food to serve four.

little enough short

---

19. The **scent** of the roses was very sweet.

color smell petals

---

20. Please **allow** me to take you to dinner.

let have love

21. You may **exit** by the stage door.

come leave listen

---

22. The story he **told** was amazing.

shouted asked related

---

23. The **container** fell off the table.

crayon box mirror

---

24. The **lid** of the bottle is broken.

handle top neck

---

25. His boss gave him a raise in **salary.**

wages taxes groceries

---

26. Her **work** was to file cards.

job destiny hope

---

27. The motor had an **oily** feel to it.

dry greasy bad

---

28. Did you finish all your **chores**?

salad papers tasks

---

29. Please **excuse** me.

expose pardon understand

---

30. The **youngsters** were playing on the swings.

infants people children

---

31. Spiders **frighten** me.

hate scare love

32. Please **shut** the door.

close lock open

---

33. Do you **understand** the directions?

read alleviate comprehend

---

34. It's cold outside; I need my **jacket.**

boots coat mittens

---

35. He **drank** the milk very quickly.

sucked swallowed solidified

---

36. She had a **fever** of 101 degrees.

temperature hot symptom

---

37. **Since** the library was closed, I went home.

After When Because

---

38. I can't **grip** the ball very well.

turn grasp drop

---

39. The **cost** of clothing is very high.

quality price inventory

---

40. My left shoulder **aches.**

hurts twitches itches

Target Area 1: Synonyms, Exercise 3

DIRECTIONS: Write a word that means the same or almost the same as the word given.

EXAMPLE: big *large*

1. handsome ______
2. selfish ______
3. wealthy ______
4. baby ______
5. pebble ______
6. underneath ______
7. howdy ______
8. misplace ______
9. hare ______
10. rifle ______
11. ill ______
12. grimy ______
13. feeble ______
14. noisy ______
15. speedy ______
16. physician ______
17. angry ______
18. interrogate ______
19. speak ______
20. recall ______
21. concrete ______
22. bigoted ______
23. quarrel ______
24. tense ______
25. assist ______
26. naughty ______
27. abdomen ______
28. terminate ______
29. boast ______
30. lawful ______
31. peaceful ______
32. sofa ______
33. battle ______
34. stupid ______
35. possess ______
36. weary ______

DIRECTIONS: Circle the word below each phrase that means the opposite of the word in dark type.

EXAMPLE: **Big** is the opposite of

large little heavy

1. **Hot** is the opposite of

   warm cold chilly

2. **Fast** is the opposite of

   trolling slow lackadaisical

3. **Angry** is the opposite of

   sad happy pleasant

4. **Peace** is the opposite of

   quiet piece war

5. **Brave** is the opposite of

   boisterous cowardly shy

6. **Dark** is the opposite of

   murky evening light

7. **Easy** is the opposite of

   intelligent hard above

8. **Dirty** is the opposite of

   clean oven ashen

9. **Sad** is the opposite of

   mad happy alarmed

10. **White** is the opposite of

yellow red black

---

11. **Smile** is the opposite of

laugh happy frown

---

12. **Run** is the opposite of

chase jog walk

---

13. **Love** is the opposite of

hate like emotion

---

14. **Messy** is the opposite of

dirty soldiers clean

---

15. **Begin** is the opposite of

start end middle

---

16. **Father** is the opposite of

mother dad infant

---

17. **Hold** is the opposite of

handle turn drop

---

18. **Send** is the opposite of

receive take letter

---

19. **Open** is the opposite of

close abduct leave

---

20. **Night** is the opposite of

evening day lightning

21. **Alone** is the opposite of

together meet after

---

22. **Adult** is the opposite of

male grownup child

---

23. **Succeed** is the opposite of

find fail donate

---

24. **Awake** is the opposite of

asleep arise apart

---

25. **Lightning** is the opposite of

hail weather thunder

---

26. **Yesterday** is the opposite of

today weekend Tuesday

---

27. **Off** is the opposite of

under on over

---

28. **Fat** is the opposite of

cute chubby thin

---

29. **In** is the opposite of

around out off

---

30. **Old** is the opposite of

antique worn new

---

31. **Stand** is the opposite of

sit walking sand

32. **Healthy** is the opposite of

sick tired lazy

---

33. **Tense** is the opposite of

calm sincere warm

---

34. **Mountain** is the opposite of

road valley hill

---

35. **Occupied** is the opposite of

eliminated outside vacant

---

36. **Up** is the opposite of

above down between

---

37. **Ride** is the opposite of

walk linger skip

---

38. **High** is the opposite of

big above low

---

39. **Over** is the opposite of

in under behind

---

40. **Small** is the opposite of

average wee large

---

41. **Even** is the opposite of

same odd subtract

---

42. **Come** is the opposite of

go sit allow

43. **Left** is the opposite of

middle right hand

---

44. **Hard** is the opposite of

tight soft puffy

---

45. **Wet** is the opposite of

slimy dry swollen

---

46. **Rise** is the opposite of

up fall midpoint

---

47. **Antonym** is the opposite of

pseudonym synonym homonym

---

48. **Take** is the opposite of

token give send

---

49. **Answer** is the opposite of

add right question

---

50. **Vertical** is the opposite of

slanted crooked horizontal

Target Area 1: Antonyms, Exercise 2

DIRECTIONS: Circle the word below the sentence that means the opposite of the word in dark type.

EXAMPLE: The horse looked very **big** next to the child.

large (little) nice

1. Look **under** the books for the newspaper.

   behind above beneath

---

2. He **loosened** his tie after the meeting.

   tightened removed tied

---

3. That man is very **tall.**

   short heavy big

---

4. It'll be easy to carry the **lightest** box.

   darkest heaviest biggest

---

5. Say **hello** to my new neighbors.

   howdy good-bye thank you

---

6. Why are there so **few** people here?

   many excited happy

---

7. Don't forget to **add** the tax to the total.

   include subtract eliminate

---

8. It's no use to **cry** over spilled milk.

   lament laugh hiccup

---

9. The weather today is **sunny.**

   cloudy rainbow dry

10. Let's take the **narrowest** path through the woods.

shortest widest sandiest

---

11. **I lost** my wallet.

misplaced bought found

---

12. Her hair is very **long** and silky.

clean short styled

---

13. Come **inside** and see our new furniture.

outside together hopping

---

14. Good **morning** to you.

weeds afternoon tomorrow

---

15. I'm glad you **arrived** on time.

attended left came

---

16. The band **often** plays on weekends.

seldom music always

---

17. We are only as **old** as we feel.

heavy young careful

---

18. The lights in the restaurant were very **bright.**

dim old large

---

19. The sea looked very **calm.**

balmy sweet rough

---

20. I baked a cake in the **square** pan.

oblong round glass

21. My **brother** looks like my father.

uncle sister mother

---

22. The mattress was very **soft.**

smooth hard fuzzy

---

23. **No,** you may not go to the movies.

maybe yes okay

---

24. Does he **work** in the factory?

play labor live

---

25. His mother **scolded** him for taking the cookies.

hit liked praised

---

26. The jury decided he was **guilty.**

tired innocent pretty

---

27. Was the **winter** very cold?

spring summer fall

---

28. I bought a **new** car.

used brown good

---

29. May I **borrow** your book?

keep lend read

---

30. The cherries were very **sweet.**

big juicy sour

---

31. Where is the **back** door of the house?

rear front porch

32. The **men** must be joking.

we women I

---

33. The chocolate sauce was very **thin.**

runny thick flavorful

---

34. **Save** your money.

deposit cash spend

---

35. My assumption was **false.**

true forthright opinionated

---

36. The laundry was **clean.**

washed dirty old

---

37. They were standing **apart.**

together tall up

---

38. The directions are **easy** to understand.

written simple difficult

---

39. This road is very **narrow.**

scenic bumpy wide

---

40. She was eager to **start** her work.

stop begin show

Target Area 1: Antonyms, Exercise 3

DIRECTIONS: Write a word that means the opposite of the word listed.

EXAMPLE: big *little*

1. rich ______
2. female ______
3. nephew ______
4. raise ______
5. bottom ______
6. careless ______
7. mine ______
8. wrong ______
9. beautiful ______
10. cool ______
11. rude ______
12. palace ______
13. push ______
14. pro ______
15. float ______
16. uncle ______
17. different ______
18. floor ______
19. daily ______
20. asleep ______
21. idle ______
22. friend ______
23. spring ______
24. past ______
25. early ______
26. nothing ______
27. whisper ______
28. wise ______
29. crooked ______
30. buy ______
31. horizontal ______
32. child ______
33. winner ______
34. attic ______
35. hate ______
36. strong ______

Target Area 1: Homonyms, Exercise

DIRECTIONS: Draw a line from the word on the left to the word or words on the right that describe it.

EXAMPLE:

horse	a raspy voice
hoarse	an animal

1. pain	ache	10. dye	pass away
pane	window part	die	tint
2. peek	highest point	11. plane	not fancy
peak	sneak a glance	plain	aircraft
3. tale	appendage	12. ate	had a meal
tail	story	eight	a number
4. rap	to knock	13. sun	opposite of moon
wrap	to tie up	son	opposite of daughter
5. hole	entire thing	14. new	had knowledge of
whole	empty place	knew	not old
6. waist	middle of the body	15. won	came in first
waste	material that's not needed	one	a number
7. week	not strong	16. ant	a relative
weak	seven days	aunt	an insect
8. stair	gaze at	17. reel	fishing gear
stare	step	real	not fake
9. brake	stop	18. weight	stay
break	destroy	wait	pounds

19.	whale	a large fish
	wail	cry and scream
20.	male	a boy
	mail	letters
21.	bough	bend from the waist
	bow	a branch on a tree
22.	fir	type of tree
	fur	covering on animals
23.	flour	found in a garden
	flower	found in a kitchen
24.	hall	passageway
	haul	carry
25.	feat	accomplishment
	feet	appendages
26.	bawled	without hair
	bald	cried
27.	suede	moved gently
	swayed	material
28.	hoarse	an animal
	horse	voice quality
29.	him	that man
	hymn	church song
30.	hire	farther up
	higher	employ
31.	aid	help
	aide	a person who helps
32.	bear	not covered
	bare	an animal
33.	stake	a piece of wood
	steak	a piece of meat
34.	lie	recline
	lye	a chemical
35.	hoes	uses a tool
	hose	garden tool
36.	pause	animal feet
	paws	take a break
37.	sundae	a dessert
	Sunday	a day
38.	quartz	rock
	quarts	measurement

Target Area 1: Homonyms, Exercise 2

DIRECTIONS: From the words above the sentences, select the correct word and fill in the blanks in the sentences.

EXAMPLE: arc ark

The arc ________ of the circle was cut.

Noah had many animals on his ark ________ .

1. ail ale

We had a glass of ________ before dinner.

If you don't get enough vitamins, you may ________ later.

---

2. build billed

The family will ________ a new house next year.

The family was ________ by the doctor's office.

---

3. urn earn

I ________ $4.00 an hour.

Put the flowers in the ________ .

---

4. creak creek

The water was clear blue in the ________ .

I heard the stairs ________ .

---

5. fined find

She was ________ for littering.

She could not ________ a four leaf clover.

---

6. seller cellar

He was a ________ of insurance.

Check the furnace in the ________ .

7. idle idol

The young boy's ____________________ was Superman.

He was ____________________ because he didn't feel like working.

---

8. told tolled

The bell ____________________ at six o'clock.

The woman ____________________ me her name.

---

9. sum some

The ____________________ of the numbers was 12.

____________________ of the numbers were missing.

---

10. lone loan

It was the ____________________ horse in the field.

The bank arranged a ____________________ so we could pay for the house.

---

11. threw through

The ball went ____________________ the window.

I ____________________ the ball at the window.

---

12. clothes close

I bought some new ____________________ .

____________________ the door when you leave.

---

13. sight site

The ____________________ of the picnic is near a stream.

The food for the picnic was a ____________________ to see.

---

14. grate great

Will you ____________________ the cheese for me?

George Washington was a ____________________ man.

15. no know

I don't ________________ of anyone who can fix it.

There is ________________ man here who can fix it.

---

16. toad toed

The ________________ is a web ________________ creature.

The ________________ is a small creature.

---

17. aye eye

Everyone in favor should say ________________ .

Please close your right ________________ .

---

18. in inn

The ________________ is full.

No one is ________________ the hotel.

We stayed ________________ the ________________ .

---

19. fare fair

Pay the ________________ before you get on the bus.

We spent the day at the ________________ .

---

20. red read

Have you ________________ the book?

Have you seen the ________________ book?

---

21. or ore

Either you ________________ I should attend the meeting.

The copper ________________ deposits are underground.

---

22. bread bred

Pass the ________________ and butter.

Good table manners show you are well ________________ .

23. carrots carats

The diamond weighs fourteen ________________ .

The rabbit ate fourteen ________________ .

---

24. sword soared

The plane ________________ over the town.

The man was polishing his ________________ .

---

25. road rode

The ________________ was full of potholes.

He ________________ with me to town.

They ________________ down the ________________ toward town.

---

26. right write rite

I want to make a ________________ turn on Maple Street.

I want to see the ________________ of graduation.

I want to ________________ to my congressman.

---

27. to two too

It was ________________ much money.

It was money ________________ go ________________ charity.

It was ________________ dollars a ticket.

---

28. they're their there

________________ going to play tennis on Saturday.

________________ playing tennis over ________________ .

________________ tennis game was not very good.

29. sew so sow

________________ the corn and peas.

________________ the skirt and blouse.

________________ what?.

---

30. sent cent scent

The flowers had a pleasant ________________ .

I don't have one ________________ to my name.

She ________________ all her clothes to the Salvation Army.

---

31. rain rein reign

Pull on the horse's ________________ .

The ________________ was coming down very hard.

The Queen will ________________ until she dies.

---

32. for fore four

The golfer yelled "________________" when he hit the ball.

The golfer hit ________________ balls.

The golfer played ________________ five hours

be-________________ he finished.

---

33. preys praise prays

The minister ________________ for the people of his congregation.

The tiger ________________ on small animals.

You should receive ________________ for a job well done.

---

34. vein vane vain

The weather ________________ pointed south.

Blood flows through our ________________ (s).

It didn't do any good: it was all in ________________ .

Target Area 1: Homonyms, Exercise 3

DIRECTIONS: Write a sentence using each of the following words correctly.

EXAMPLE: horse I have never ridden a horse.

hoarse His voice was hoarse from yelling at the game.

1. flee ____________________

   flea ____________________

2. blue ____________________

   blew ____________________

3. pare ____________________

   pear ____________________

4. foul ____________________

   fowl ____________________

5. buy ______________________________

____

by ______________________________

____

6. seam ______________________________

____

seem ______________________________

____

7. night ______________________________

____

knight ______________________________

____

8. sale ______________________________

____

sail ______________________________

____

9. heal ______________________________

____

heel ______________________________

____

10. led ______________________________

____

lead ______________________________

____

11. seen ______________________________

____

scene ______________________________

____

12. way ______________________________

____

weigh ______________________________

____

13. our ______________________________

____

hour ______________________________

____

14. hare ______________________________

____

hair ______________________________

____

15. poll ______________________________

____

pole ______________________________

____

16. dough ______________________________

____

doe ______________________________

____

17. grown ______________________________

____

groan ______________________________

____

18. piece ______________________________

____

peace ______________________________

____

19. tied ______________________________

____

tide ______________________________

____

20. wade ______________________________

____

weighed ______________________________

____

Target Area 1: Homonyms, Exercise 4

DIRECTIONS: Write one sentence using both words.

EXAMPLE: hoarse, horse

I was hoarse from yelling at the horse race.

1. wood, would

2. herd, heard

3. beet, beat

4. hear, here

5. not, knot

6. bee, be

7. nose, knows

8. bored, board

9. dear, deer

10. roll, role ________________________________

____

11. acts, axe ________________________________

____

12. aisle, I'll ________________________________

____

13. aloud, allowed ____________________________

____

14. gilt, guilt ________________________________

____

15. made, maid ______________________________

____

16. passed, past ______________________________

____

17. ring, wring ______________________________

____

18. band, banned ____________________________

____

19. eerie, Erie ________________________________

____

20. Yule, you'll ______________________________

____

Target Area 1: Vocabulary, Exercise 1

DIRECTIONS: One word in each **right** column best fits each word in the column to the **left** of it. Put the letter of that word in the blank next to the word it fits.

EXAMPLE:

goalpost __b__	a. ball
hockey __c__	b. football
base __a__	c. puck

strike ____	a. attorney	orchid ____	a. ligament
rose ____	b. dinner	cinnamon ____	b. nest
chicken ____	c. thorn	rifle ____	c. light
lawyer ____	d. actress	bird ____	d. river
gloves ____	e. 1/2	muscle ____	e. gun
onion ____	f. spare	battle ____	f. gate
half ____	g. oven	college ____	g. flower
socks ____	h. mittens	dollar ____	h. money
supper ____	i. %	lake ____	i. gas
stove ____	j. poultry	lamp ____	j. fight
professor ____	k. odor	fuel ____	k. hatchet
fingers ____	l. teacher	steel ____	l. spice
actor ____	m. town	axe ____	m. forest
village ____	n. stockings	fence ____	n. metal
percent ____	o. thumb	trees ____	o. university

pickle ____	a. andirons	smoke ____	a. eyes
blackboard ____	b. auto	drink ____	b. door
foot ____	c. saddle	sweep ____	c. cake
relative ____	d. toe	bake ____	d. cigarette
teeth ____	e. wick	weigh ____	e. mountain
candle ____	f. cucumber	blink ____	f. airplane
thermometer ____	g. oar	dial ____	g. floor
sedan ____	h. uncle	fly ____	h. lawn
lawn ____	i. temperature	climb ____	i. water
fireplace ____	j. sill	sing ____	j. scale
frozen ____	k. chalk	knock ____	k. race
rowboat ____	l. hoe	mow ____	l. song
horse ____	m. grass	sharpen ____	m. phone
window ____	n. ice	run ____	n. parade
rake ____	o. jaw	march ____	o. pencil

shave ______	a.	boat
boil ______	b.	letter
bark ______	c.	ball
vote ______	d.	water
preach ______	e.	shovel
write ______	f.	car
sit ______	g.	whiskers
run ______	h.	numbers
add ______	i.	sermon
drive ______	j.	field
dig ______	k.	dog
lock ______	l.	chair
sail ______	m.	election
plow ______	n.	key
throw ______	o.	race

fruit ______	a.	begonia
furniture ______	b.	mosquito
clothing ______	c.	desk
jewelry ______	d.	October
month ______	e.	leopard
country ______	f.	peach
shape ______	g.	sparrow
animal ______	h.	dishwasher
insect ______	i.	watch
illness ______	j.	rectangle
appliance ______	k.	celery
sport ______	l.	hockey
vegetable ______	m.	sweater
flower ______	n.	cancer
bird ______	o.	India

Target Area 1: Vocabulary, Exercise 2

DIRECTIONS: Pick a word on the right that means the same or almost the same as the word on the left. Put the letter of that word in the blank, next to the word on the left.

EXAMPLE:

huge b	a. begin
tiny c	b. big
start a	c. small

rubbish ____	a. often
pottery ____	b. burn
frequently ____	c. frown
umbrella ____	d. pig
prankster ____	e. fighter
scowl ____	f. garbage
twig ____	g. purse
scorch ____	h. visitor
gaze ____	i. parasol
pocketbook ____	j. Satan
warrior ____	k. ceramics
devil ____	l. branch
guest ____	m. couch
hog ____	n. joker
sofa ____	o. stare

always ____	a. evil
trousers ____	b. mad
artificial ____	c. tardy
insane ____	d. pants
attempt ____	e. cent
sinful ____	f. try
wed ____	g. thin
sack ____	h. forever
penny ____	i. location
build ____	j. bag
late ____	k. fake
mimic ____	l. construct
site ____	m. marry
slender ____	n. allow
let ____	o. imitate
rubdown ____	p. massage

dry _____	a. petty
height _____	b. complain
protest _____	c. confused
easy _____	d. arid
rely _____	e. motto
adequate _____	f. reduce
bewildered _____	g. depend
meaningful _____	h. significant
trivial _____	i. jealous
recover _____	j. altitude
discount _____	k. pail
immense _____	l. sufficient
envious _____	m. simple
slogan _____	n. colossal
bucket _____	o. recuperate

Target Area 1: Vocabulary, Exercise 3

DIRECTIONS: Pick the best definition for the word on the left from the words on the right. Put the letter of the definition next to the word it defines.

EXAMPLE:

stem __b__	a. something to drink
boat __c__	b. part of a plant
lemonade __a__	c. a sailing vessel

caterpillar _____	a. without prejudice
hour _____	b. the right amount
enough _____	c. to look for
prank _____	d. flavoring for food
ground _____	e. young butterfly
impartial _____	f. insect that eats wood
tremble _____	g. four-sided solid shape
cube _____	h. surface of the earth
nostrils _____	i. large, stately home
wig _____	j. mischievous trick
search _____	k. not alike
mansion _____	l. sixty minutes
different _____	m. openings in the nose
seasoning _____	n. shake with fear
termite _____	o. covering for the head

detour _____	a. lower part of the leg
crooked _____	b. home for the Eskimo
starve _____	c. able to be heard
yacht _____	d. not straight
audible _____	e. more than one
whisper _____	f. roundabout way to get somewhere
rouge _____	g. talk softly
chin _____	h. hair on the face
shin _____	i. stay away from
width _____	j. cosmetic for the cheeks
plural _____	k. large luxurious boat
igloo _____	l. distance across something
avoid _____	m. suffer because of hunger
obey _____	n. do what you're told to
whiskers _____	o. lower part of the face

saddle _____	a. instrument telling direction
prevent _____	b. mix up
coward _____	c. bring from another country
import _____	d. keep from happening
beard _____	e. part of an auto wheel
thigh _____	f. two of a kind
compass _____	g. vacation spot
discuss _____	h. put in a bank
tire _____	i. unexpected event
deposit _____	j. worn by a horse
pair _____	k. part of a leg
confuse _____	l. wooden spike
stake _____	m. facial hair
resort _____	n. person who is not brave
surprise _____	o. talk about

manicure _____	a. Italian appetizer
income _____	b. skin irritation
rash _____	c. without shoes or socks
anthem _____	d. last car on a train
candidate _____	e. ten year period
solution _____	f. someone running for office
caboose _____	g. a drinking container
bandage _____	h. care for the nails
antipasto _____	i. class for small children
decade _____	j. answer to a problem
mug _____	k. national song
hem _____	l. border of clothing
barefoot _____	m. wound covering
island _____	n. land surrounded by water
kindergarten _____	o. money earned

photographer _____	a. one who works with wood
maid _____	b. one who fills prescriptions
physician _____	c. one who helps sick people
banker _____	d. one who cooks
mathematician _____	e. one who delivers letters
receptionist _____	f. one who sews
dentist _____	g. one who serves in a restaurant
chauffeur _____	h. one who is concerned with the teeth
chef _____	i. one who greets people
druggist _____	j. one who works with money
mailman _____	k. one who takes pictures
plumber _____	l. one who works with numbers
carpenter _____	m. one who is paid to clean house
waitress _____	n. one who fixes pipes
seamstress _____	o. one who drives people to places

Target Area 1: Vocabulary, Exercise 4

DIRECTIONS: On another sheet of paper write an explanation of what each of the following words means. Do not use a dictionary.

EXAMPLE: Define **purple.** Purple is a color that is a combination of red and blue.

1. Define **rainbow.**
2. Define **difficult.**
3. Define **county.**
4. Define **broken.**
5. Define **screwdriver.**
6. Define **reward.**
7. Define **conference.**
8. Define **frame.**
9. Define **stockholder.**
10. Define **equator.**
11. Define **postpone.**
12. Define **Halloween.**
13. Define **tonsils.**
14. Define **minute.**
15. Define **explosion.**
16. Define **coupon.**
17. Define **taxi.**
18. Define **honest.**
19. Define **decision.**
20. Define **omelette.**
21. Define **foreign.**
22. Define **veterinarian.**
23. Define **flashlight.**
24. Define **population.**
25. Define **tourist.**
26. Define **suffocate.**
27. Define **movie.**
28. Define **buzzard.**
29. Define **acre.**
30. Define **dimples.**
31. Define **emotion.**
32. Define **trunk.**
33. Define **inflation.**
34. Define **sophisticated.**
35. Define **arrest.**
36. Define **wharf.**
37. Define **democracy.**
38. Define **handle.**
39. Define **promotion.**
40. Define **porch.**

Target Area 1: Word Formation, Exercise 1

DIRECTIONS: Add one or more letters to the listed letters so that words are formed.

EXAMPLE:

so *da* ______	so *cks* ______
so *ur* ______	so *n* ______
so *metimes* ______	so *uth* ______

1. ba ______	4. pe ______
ba ______	pe ______
ba ______	pe ______
ba ______	pe ______
ba ______	pe ______
ba ______	pe ______
2. ch ______	5. ex ______
ch ______	ex ______
ch ______	ex ______
ch ______	ex ______
ch ______	ex ______
ch ______	ex ______
3. st ______	6. co ______
st ______	co ______
st ______	co ______
st ______	co ______
st ______	co ______
st ______	co ______

7. sh ______________________
sh ______________________
sh ______________________
sh ______________________
sh ______________________
sh ______________________

8. ki ______________________
ki ______________________
ki ______________________
ki ______________________
ki ______________________
ki ______________________

9. tr ______________________
tr ______________________
tr ______________________
tr ______________________
tr ______________________
tr ______________________

10. be ______________________
be ______________________
be ______________________
be ______________________
be ______________________
be ______________________

11. qu ______________________
qu ______________________
qu ______________________
qu ______________________
qu ______________________
qu ______________________

12. ar ______________________
ar ______________________
ar ______________________
ar ______________________
ar ______________________
ar ______________________

13. bl ______________________
bl ______________________
bl ______________________
bl ______________________
bl ______________________
bl ______________________

14. we ______________________
we ______________________
we ______________________
we ______________________
we ______________________
we ______________________

15. in ____________________

in ____________________

in ____________________

in ____________________

in ____________________

in ____________________

Directions: Continue as above, but insert the beginning letter(s).

---

16. ____________________ art

____________________ art

____________________ art

____________________ art

____________________ art

____________________ art

17. ____________________ op

____________________ op

____________________ op

____________________ op

____________________ op

____________________ op

18. ____________________ ack

____________________ ack

____________________ ack

____________________ ack

____________________ ack

____________________ ack

19. ____________________ ime

____________________ ime

____________________ ime

____________________ ime

____________________ ime

____________________ ime

20. ____________________ ig

____________________ ig

____________________ ig

____________________ ig

____________________ ig

____________________ ig

21. ____________________ oat

____________________ oat

____________________ oat

____________________ oat

____________________ oat

____________________ oat

22. ______________________ ar
______________________ ar
______________________ ar
______________________ ar
______________________ ar
______________________ ar

23. ______________________ sh
______________________ sh
______________________ sh
______________________ sh
______________________ sh
______________________ sh

24. ______________________ y
______________________ y
______________________ y
______________________ y
______________________ y
______________________ y

25. ______________________ tion
______________________ tion
______________________ tion
______________________ tion
______________________ tion
______________________ tion

26. ______________________ ment
______________________ ment
______________________ ment
______________________ ment
______________________ ment
______________________ ment

27. ______________________ able
______________________ able
______________________ able
______________________ able
______________________ able
______________________ able

28. ______________________ ing
______________________ ing
______________________ ing
______________________ ing
______________________ ing
______________________ ing

29. ______________________ ch
______________________ ch
______________________ ch
______________________ ch
______________________ ch
______________________ ch

30. ______________ er
______________ er
______________ er
______________ er
______________ er
______________ er

Directions: Continue as above, but insert at least one letter on each side of the letter given.

31. ______ pa r ty ______	34. ______ st ______
______ r ______	______ st ______
______ r ______	______ st ______
______ r ______	______ st ______
______ r ______	______ st ______
______ r ______	______ st ______
32. ______ u ______	35. ______ th ______
______ u ______	______ th ______
______ u ______	______ th ______
______ u ______	______ th ______
______ u ______	______ th ______
______ u ______	______ th ______
33. ______ n ______	36. ______ bb ______
______ n ______	______ bb ______
______ n ______	______ bb ______
______ n ______	______ bb ______
______ n ______	______ bb ______
______ n ______	______ bb ______

37. ______ ch ______
______ ch ______
______ ch ______
______ ch ______
______ ch ______
______ ch ______

38. ______ m ______
______ m ______
______ m ______
______ m ______
______ m ______
______ m ______

39. ______ tt ______
______ tt ______
______ tt ______
______ tt ______
______ tt ______
______ tt ______

40. ______ oa ______
______ oa ______
______ oa ______
______ oa ______
______ oa ______
______ oa ______

41. ______ ee ______
______ ee ______
______ ee ______
______ ee ______
______ ee ______
______ ee ______

42. ______ sh ______
______ sh ______
______ sh ______
______ sh ______
______ sh ______
______ sh ______

43. ______ oo ______
______ oo ______
______ oo ______
______ oo ______
______ oo ______
______ oo ______

44. ______ at ______
______ at ______
______ at ______
______ at ______
______ at ______
______ at ______

Target Area 1: Word Formation, Exercise 2

DIRECTIONS: Think of as many words as you can that **rhyme** with each word listed and write them on another sheet of paper. It might help to write down the alphabet as well.

EXAMPLE: cap *chap, flap, lap, clap, map, nap, trap, strap, snap, wrap, gap, scrap*

1. pot
2. late
3. cake
4. snore
5. brain
6. spent
7. black
8. west
9. rude
10. tin
11. stay
12. split
13. an
14. steed
15. mean
16. think
17. thrill
18. rat
19. queer
20. glue
21. sag
22. your
23. said
24. spell
25. cheek
26. square
27. streak
28. trip
29. thrust
30. rolled

Target Area 1: Categorizing, Exercise 1

DIRECTIONS: From the list of words at the bottom of the page, choose the words that fit under the correct heading. Cross out the words in the list as you use them. Each word is used once.

EXAMPLE:

Animals	Birds
cat	*robin*
dog	*cardinal*
horse	*crow*

~~cat~~ ~~dog~~ ~~crow~~
~~robin~~ ~~cardinal~~ ~~horse~~

a. Things you hear but don't ride

______
______
______
______
______
______

b. Things you ride

______
______
______
______
______
______

c. Things you smell but don't taste

______
______
______
______
______
______

d. Things you taste

______
______
______
______
______
______

carousel	noise	whistles	skunks
perfume	train	applause	laughter
gumdrops	butter	cookies	plane
liver	buzzing	flowers	rubbing alcohol
sirens	smoke	corn	tomatoes
bicycle	horse	leaking gas	motorcycle

a. Words connected with winter	b. Words connected with summer
______	______
______	______
______	______
______	______
______	______
______	______

c. Things made from flour	d. Things out of the ocean
______	______
______	______
______	______
______	______
______	______
______	______

seahorse	sunny and warm	pancakes	blizzards
bread	cookies	cold	fresh flowers
gravy	coral	sunglasses	jellyfish
hot	frost	snowy	rolls
icicles	green	pastry	sunburn
shells	algae	salt water	boots

a. Containers	b. Cooking terms
__________	__________
__________	__________
__________	__________
__________	__________
__________	__________
__________	__________

c. Halloween terms	d. Telephone terms
__________	__________
__________	__________
__________	__________
__________	__________
__________	__________
__________	__________

boil	candy	crates	area code
dial tone	fry	ghosts	simmer
trick or treat	cartons	operator	envelopes
costumes	receiver	suitcases	scald
bottles	witches	jack-o-lanterns	hello
extension	bake	broil	drawers

a. Things to make with apples	b. Things to take on a picnic other than food
__________	__________
__________	__________
__________	__________
__________	__________
__________	__________
__________	__________
c. Ways of communicating	**d. Shiny things**
__________	__________
__________	__________
__________	__________
__________	__________
__________	__________
__________	__________

basket	strudel	letter	cobbler
pie	dumplings	chrome	paper plates
mirrors	charcoal	tablecloth	morse code
plastic silverware	talking	gestures	cider
intercom	napkins	sun	silver buckle
tinsel	sauce	silver dollar	telegram

a. Words of three syllables

____

____

____

____

____

____

b. Words ending in **-ble**

____

____

____

____

____

____

c. Words beginning with **wh-**

____

____

____

____

____

____

d. Words of four syllables

____

____

____

____

____

____

predominant	dribble	table	indigestible
wholesale	hysteria	Arkansas	macaroni
cable	whisk	lieutenant	submarine
rigorous	arrangement	negotiate	wheat
bubble	who	whirlwind	disagreeable
whiskey	speculation	obnoxious	territory

a. Things to walk on

____
____
____
____
____
____

b. Things to live in

____
____
____
____
____
____

c. Baseball terms

____
____
____
____
____
____

d. Football terms

____
____
____
____
____
____

igloo	goal post	tent	umpire
touchdown	tackle	gravel	condominium
out	inning	foul	1st and 10
sidewalk	dog house	quarterback	dugout
tightrope	grass	hut	carpet
trailer	strike	beach	field goal

a. Planets	b. Gasoline companies
__________	__________
__________	__________
__________	__________
__________	__________
__________	__________
__________	__________
c. State capitals	**d. Rivers**
__________	__________
__________	__________
__________	__________
__________	__________
__________	__________
__________	__________

Seine	Richmond	Nile	Raleigh
Augusta	Pluto	Shell	Jupiter
Montgomery	Texaco	Mobil	Venus
Mississippi	Yangtze	Sacramento	Atlantic Richfield
Mars	Gulf	Boston	Amazon
Standard	Swanee	Neptune	Saturn

Target Area 1: Categorizing, Exercise 2

DIRECTIONS: Some letters are missing in the following words. Fill in the missing letters to form words to fit the categories listed.

EXAMPLE: **Ways to cook eggs**

s c r a m b l e d　　f r i e d

p o a c h e d　　o m e l e t t e

h a r d b o i l e d

1. **Colors**

r ___ d

b l ___ ___

w ___ ___ t ___

p ___ n k

b l ___ ___ k

o r ___ ___ g ___

g ___ ___ e n

___ ___ l l ___ w

2. **Articles on the dinner table**

p l ___ ___ e

k ___ ___ f ___

s ___ l t

g ___ ___ s s

f ___ r k

___ p o ___ n

n a ___ k ___ ___

p ___ p p ___ r

3. **Wild animals**

b ___ ___ r

___ e o p ___ ___ d

c ___ u g ___ r

e ___ e ___ ___ a ___ t

t ___ g ___ r

g ___ r ___ l l a

___ ___ r ___ f f ___

l i ___ ___

4. **Appliances**

s t ___ v ___

v ___ ___ u u ___

t e l ___ v ___ s i ___ n

d ___ s h w ___ ___ h ___ r

d ___ y ___ r

t ___ ___ s t ___ r

c ___ n ___ p ___ n ___ r

f ___ ___ ___ z ___ r

5. **Baked goods**

p i ___

e c l ___ ___ ___

c ___ k ___

d ___ ___ g h ___ u ___

___ o o k ___ ___

c ___ p c ___ k ___

b r ___ w ___ ___ ___

___ ___ e a d

6. **Things found in the ocean**

a l ___ a e

f ___ ___ h

___ h ___ l e

s ___ ___ n g e

___ ___ l

o c ___ ___ p u s

s h ___ ___ k s

___ y s t ___ ___ s

7. **Measurements**

t ___ b l ___ s ___ ___ ___ n

g ___ l l ___ n

p ___ n t

q u ___ ___ t

___ e t ___ r

___ ___ a s p o ___ ___

o u ___ c ___

p ___ ___ n d

8. **Nuts**

___ ___ s h e w

p ___ ___ n u t

p ___ s t ___ ___ h ___ o

w ___ ___ n ___ t

___ c ___ r n

p ___ c ___ n

___ l m ___ ___ d

c h ___ ___ t ___ u t

9. **Internal organs**

l ___ v ___ r

k ___ d n ___ ___

h e ___ r ___

s ___ ___ m ___ c h

v ___ ___ n s

b ___ a ___ n

___ p p ___ n d ___ x

l ___ n ___ s

10. **Airplane terms**

a ___ r p ___ r ___

p ___ l ___ t

w ___ n g ___

s t ___ w ___ ___ ___ ___ s s

b ___ g g ___ g ___

t ___ ___ k ___ t

j ___ t

t ___ r m ___ n ___ l

11. **Cheeses**

___ w ___ s s

A ___ e r ___ c a ___

___ a r m e ___ a n

___ o z a ___ ___ l l a

c ___ e d ___ a r

c r ___ ___ m

r ___ c o t ___ a

C ___ l b y

12. **Feelings**

s ___ ___

___ ___ p p ___

___ x c ___ t ___ ___

a ___ ___ r y

j ___ y f ___ l

n ___ r v ___ ___ ___

___ ___ l m

s c ___ r ___ d

13. **World capitals**

P a ___ ___ s

R ___ m ___

M ___ s c ___ ___

L o ___ d ___ ___

___ a d r ___ d

P ___ k ___ n g

___ o ___ o ___ u l u

O ___ t ___ w a

14. **Vegetables**

___ ___ r n

___ o ___ a ___ o ___ s

___ r ___ c c ___ l ___

___ e t t ___ c ___

b e ___ ___ s

___ q u ___ ___ h

___ s p a r ___ g u ___

o ___ ___ o n

15. **Metals**

___ r ___ n

s t ___ ___ l

c ___ p p ___ ___

z ___ ___ c

___ ___ l v ___ r

p l ___ t ___ n ___ m

g ___ l ___

l ___ a d

16. **Things you can cut**

b ___ e ___ d

r ___ b ___ o n

p a p ___ ___

___ i n ___ ___ ___ n a i l s

h ___ ___ r

c ___ k ___

w ___ r e

___ r ___ s s

17. **Things you find in a library**

___ o o ___ s

___ a r ___ c a t ___ l ___ g

t a b ___ ___ s

___ i b ___ a ___ i a n

r ___ ___ o ___ d s

m ___ g a ___ i n ___ s

___ i c t ___ ___ n ___ ___ y

___ ___ e l v ___ s

18. **Things you can lock**

___ ___ o r

s ___ f ___

b r ___ e f c ___ s ___

___ e w e ___ r y ___ ___ x

___ u ___ o m ___ b i ___ e

d ___ s k

___ ___ u n k

f i l ___

19. Snacks

___ r ___ t z ___ l s

p ___ a n ___ t s

___ o ___ a ___ o

c h ___ ___ s

p ___ p ___ o ___ ___

___ ___ l k   s h ___ k ___

___ p p l ___ s

___ r ___ c k ___ r s

c ___ n d ___   b ___ r

20. Italian food

___ p ___ g h e t ___ i

a n ___ i p a ___ t o

___ a s a g n ___

m ___ n e ___ t r o n ___

___ i z ___ a

r a v ___ o l ___

s p u m ___ n i

___ a s t a

21. Materials

___ o t t ___ n

___ u ___ d e

c ___ r d ___ r ___ y

___ ___ l k

___ o o l

d ___ n ___ m

p ___ l ___ e s t ___ r

l ___ ___ t h ___ r

22. Containers

b ___ g

___ o u c h

d r ___ w e ___

___ ___ r t o n

p ___ r s ___

c r ___ t e

s h o ___   ___ ___ x

b ___ w l

23. **U.S. presidents**

___ i n c ___ l n

R ___ ___ s ___ v ___ l ___

___ a s h ___ ___ g t ___ ___

K ___ n n ___ ___ y

M ___ K ___ ___ l ___ ___

___ r u ___ a n

E ___ s ___ ___ h ___ ___ ___ ___

___ ___ f f ___ r s ___ n

24. **Fish**

h ___ l ___ b ___ t

___ u n a

___ ___ r c h

___ e d   s ___ a p ___ ___ r

c ___ d

___ a r d ___ n e ___

t r ___ ___ t

s ___ l m ___ n

25. **Occupations**

n ___ r s ___

t e ___ c h ___ ___

___ a w y ___ r

___ e c r ___ ___ a r ___

c l ___ ___ k

f ___ r ___ m ___ n

___ a ___ t r e s ___

p ___ u m b ___ r

26. **Things to watch**

b ___ ___ d s

___ e l e ___ i s ___ o ___

s ___ n s ___ t

___ o v ___ e

p a ___ ___ d e

r ___ c ___ s

b a ___ e b a ___ ___

___ l a ___ s

Target Area 1: Categorizing, Exercise 3

DIRECTIONS: On another sheet of paper, write all the words you can think of that belong in the categories listed. Try to write down at least 15 in each category.

EXAMPLE: animals *bear, dog, elephant, raccoon, monkey, lion, kangaroo, cat, beaver, giraffe, hamster, mouse, tiger, otter*

1. things to write with
2. flowers
3. tools
4. parts of a car
5. breakfast foods
6. sports
7. kinds of candies
8. things to buy in a bakery
9. words ending in **-sh**
10. words ending in **-th**
11. song titles
12. TV shows
13. things made of metal
14. actresses
15. things you buy in pairs
16. things that bake in an oven
17. cities in your state
18. occupations
19. words of two syllables
20. things made of wood
21. soups
22. European countries
23. words that describe spring
24. things you do **every** day
25. things that are soft
26. things to ride
27. streets in your area
28. famous people in history
29. actors
30. islands
31. things that come in bottles
32. kitchen utensils
33. things to buy in a drugstore
34. kinds of cars
35. things in the sky
36. furry things

Target Area 1: Abbreviations

DIRECTIONS: Write out the words for which the following initials stand.

EXAMPLE: VA *Veterans Administration*

1. USA ______
2. NBC ______
3. Ph.D. ______
4. MGM ______
5. GM ______
6. c.o.d. ______
7. YMCA ______
8. FBI ______
9. USSR ______
10. I.Q. ______
11. UN ______
12. p.m. ______
13. AAA ______
14. AT & T ______
15. IBM ______
16. VP ______
17. M.D. ______
18. NFL ______
19. AMA ______
20. UAW ______
21. qt. ______
22. atty. ______
23. Eng. ______
24. Feb. ______

25. doz. ______
26. etc. ______
27. Jr. ______
28. gal. ______
29. Mon. ______
30. ave. ______
31. Mr. ______
32. bldg. ______
33. ft. ______
34. Oct. ______
35. Capt. ______
36. misc. ______
37. c/o ______
38. Rep. ______
39. univ. ______
40. dept. ______
41. yr. ______
42. pd. ______
43. m.p.h. ______
44. Aug. ______
45. apt. ______
46. yd. ______
47. mfg. ______
48. govt. ______
49. rec'd. ______
50. St. ______

Target Area 1: Dictionary Usage, Exercise 1

DIRECTIONS: The following words will probably be unfamiliar to you, so you will need a dictionary. Write each word on a separate sheet of paper, then look up the word in the dictionary. Write a definition of each word, rewriting the dictionary definition in your own words if you can.

EXAMPLE: botanist *a botanist is a person who studie's plants.*

1. panegyric
2. cacophony
3. apocryphal
4. embrocate
5. marmoreal
6. brummagem
7. succussion
8. prurient
9. virago
10. ziggurat
11. velleity
12. piacular
13. helicoid
14. nimiety
15. grovel
16. encomium
17. deracinate
18. orison
19. bohea
20. wimble
21. asteroid
22. caisson
23. thaumaturge
24. sapor
25. truckle
26. bunco
27. rachitis
28. libidinous
29. mastic
30. viridity

Target Area 1: Dictionary Usage, Exercise 2

DIRECTIONS: You may need a dictionary for this exercise. Each sentence has several large words in it. Under each sentence there is a word you are to define. Write this definition in your own words using it in the same way as it was used in the sentence. Under the definition rewrite the sentence in your own words so that it is much easier to understand. Make sure that you replace all of the words in dark type with your own words. You may rewrite the entire sentence if you wish, as long as it means about the same thing as the first sentence.

EXAMPLE: The **gentleman** was a **botanist.**

Botanist: *someone who studies plants.*

sentence: *The man knows a great deal about plants.*

1. The **holocaust** following the earthquake was **devastating.**

   Holocaust: ______

   sentence: ______

   ______

2. Joe's **brother's wife** is a **philatelist.**

   Philatelist: ______

   sentence: ______

   ______

3. The **recalcitrant adolescent** would not **yield his position** on smoking.

   Recalcitrant: ______

   sentence: ______

   ______

4. Even though we **attempted** to **pacify** her, she was too **fastidious.**

   Fastidious: ______________________________

   sentence: ______________________________

   ____

---

5. He **repudiated** any **insinuation** that he was **obese.**

   Repudiated: ______________________________

   sentence: ______________________________

   ____

---

6. He was a **dauntless aviator.**

   Dauntless: ______________________________

   sentence: ______________________________

   ____

---

7. Their **squalid living conditions** made me **apprehensive** when I visited.

   Squalid: ______________________________

   sentence: ______________________________

   ____

---

8. Her **vivacious chatter amused** the group.

   Vivacious: ______________________________

   sentence: ______________________________

   ____

---

9. The **morose** boy refused to **grin** at the clown's **antics.**

   Morose: ______________________________

   sentence: ______________________________

   ____

10. Her **pallid** appearance made me wonder if she was **ailing.**

Pallid: ________________________

sentence: ________________________

____

---

11. The **sojourn** was pleasant, but **lengthy.**

Sojourn: ________________________

sentence: ________________________

____

---

12. The kitten **parried** the **attempts** of the dog to **romp** with her.

Parried: ________________________

sentence: ________________________

____

---

13. The **mullets** were **in abundance** near the shore line.

Mullets: ________________________

sentence: ________________________

____

---

14. His **lethargy** was obvious by the **sluggish** way that he moved.

Lethargy: ________________________

sentence: ________________________

____

---

15. Her explanation was so **lucid,** we could **visualize** the scene in our minds.

Lucid: ________________________

sentence: ________________________

____

16. The casserole was **tepid** when it **was brought to** our table.

Tepid: ______________________________

sentence: ______________________________

____

17. The **apiary** was filled with a **plethora** of hornets.

Plethora: ______________________________

sentence: ______________________________

____

18. The guest speaker entered the **postern unbeknownst** to us.

Postern: ______________________________

sentence: ______________________________

____

19. Our **itinerary** for the trip was in a state of **flux.**

Itinerary: ______________________________

sentence: ______________________________

____

20. The comedian **japed** at the audience during his **debut** at the club.

Japed: ______________________________

sentence: ______________________________

____

21. I find your **mythical** tales quite **incredible.**

Mythical: ______________________________

sentence: ______________________________

____

22. I was **disgusted** with the **paltry** appearance of the **eating establishment** and I **vowed** I would never **go back.**

Paltry: ____________________

sentence: ____________________

____

23. The **rancor** the boy had toward the class bully **compelled** him to be **sarcastic.**

Rancor: ____________________

sentence: ____________________

____

24. After some **vichyssoise,** I would like some pie **a la mode.**

Vichyssoise: ____________________

sentence: ____________________

____

25. The **canine** was stretched out in a **supine position** on the **sofa.**

Supine: ____________________

sentence: ____________________

____

26. She was **naive** about his **persistent attempts** to **woo** her.

Naive: ____________________

sentence: ____________________

____

27. The **cogent** remarks helped to **convey** the **essence** of the problem.

Cogent: ____________________

sentence: ____________________

____

28. The jury made an **erroneous** decision regarding her **criminality.**

Erroneous: ______________________________

sentence: ______________________________

____

29. Their **sojourn** into the **bucolic** countryside of New Hampshire was very **pleasant.**

Bucolic: ______________________________

sentence: ______________________________

____

30. There were so many **fallacies** in the **tale** that I feel the whole thing was **hyperbolic.**

Hyperbolic: ______________________________

sentence: ______________________________

____

31. An **incision** was made into the **tissue** above the **sternum.**

Sternum: ______________________________

sentence: ______________________________

____

32. The **patois** of the **alien** made it difficult for us to **comprehend** him.

Patois: ______________________________

sentence: ______________________________

____

33. When we attained a **quorum,** we **started** the meeting.

Quorum: ______________________________

sentence: ______________________________

____

34. She was a **patron** of the symphony and a **dilettante.**

Dilettante: ____________________

sentence: ____________________

____

35. The **attorney** had a certain **suave, sophisticated** air about him.

Suave: ____________________

sentence: ____________________

____

36. When he is **angry I avoid** him because of his **pugilistic tendencies.**

Pugilisitic: ____________________

sentence: ____________________

____

37. That man had so much **charisma I** never would have **suspected** that he dealt in **contraband goods.**

Charisma: ____________________

sentence: ____________________

____

38. Her **florid complexion** made her look **robust.**

Robust: ____________________

sentence: ____________________

____

39. Her **predecessor** thought that her **precociousness** would be an **asset** to her.

Precociousness: ____________________

sentence: ____________________

____

Target Area 2
DEVELOPMENT OF SYNTAX

Syntax is a critical component of basic communication, for the flow of language is expressed in oral and graphic syntax as ideas and thoughts develop. Target Area Two emphasizes the reestablishment of language flow and the development of sentence structure. The following exercises cover such areas as morphemic usage, punctuation, and sentence, phrase, and paragraph construction, giving the patient an opportunity to organize the various elements of language into syntactic responses.

The use of punctuation and capitalization is the focus of the first exercise. The patient must insert appropriate responses into existing sentences and then copy them. Other exercises concern the correct use of grammar. Phrase Completions ask for answers in several parts of speech; many of these questions use common expressions or well known sayings. In Sentence Construction the patient makes an original sentence from a given word or phrase, and in Paragraph Construction he expands this activity to the creation of actual paragraphs or short stories. Thus the patient gains more experience with complete expression of thought. Two exercises in the Supplementary Materials section use one word as several parts of speech and may be useful in conjunction with this target area.

The patient can and should spend considerable time on Target Area Two, as the fluent use of syntactic structures is vital to adequate communication.

M.R.

Target Area 2: Punctuation

DIRECTIONS: In the following sentences, all forms of punctuation (such as periods, capitals, commas, quotations, and question marks) have been left out. Rewrite each sentence correctly by adding any punctuation needed.

EXAMPLE: where is bob going *Where is Bob going?*

1. where do you live ____________________

2. i live in detroit mich ____________________

3. it seemed as though the time would never pass ____________________

4. it was very noisy but i really enjoyed the tour ____________________

5. my brother the one in the plaid jacket is getting married in april ____________________

6. is that a chevrolet or a buick ____________________

7. my wife has invited you and betty over for dinner friday night ____

8. i wish i could remember what i wanted to buy ____

9. today is jan 29 1976 ____

10. dick asked how are you ____

DIRECTIONS: Continue as before, but also correct any spelling errors that you notice.

11. im fine i replied ____

12. her desert had apples bannanas pineapple and kokonut in it ____

13. i dont know witch dress i should pick ____

14. after we had lunch we went to the lawndrey the hardware store the post offise and the ymca ____

15. joe namath a handsome football player will be feashured in a special tv show ______________________________

16. who do you think is the better aktress mary tyler moore or jill st john ______________________________

17. man overbored get the lifeboats the captin shouted ______________________________

18. i cant rember whether vetrins day is in may or sepember ______________________________

19. you should be able to find an artikel on canser in the journal of medecine ______________________________

20. jack linda mary don sue and i want to go horseback rideing but we dont know where the stabells are ______________________________

21. this isnt the way its supozed to look ______________________________

22. mr jones the one in the blue coat mrs black the one with the white gloves and mr mcadam are the leaders ______________________________

____

____

23. warning take only as directed by your dr at 800 am 1200 pm and 400 pm ____

____

____

24. your supposed to yell help if anythings wrong ______________

____

____

25. clark gable said to scarlet ohara frankly my dear i dont give a dam

____

____

26. jackolanterns are eazier to carve after the paulp has been removed

____

____

____

27. in order to have a compleat meal you should include a meat vege table dary product and fruit ______________________

____

____

28. will you please send in a supply order for rubber bands paper clips stapels legal pads and pencils ______________________

____

____

Target Area 2: Morphemic Usage, Exercise 1

DIRECTIONS: Circle the word(s) that best fits into the blank in the sentence.

EXAMPLE: She ________ twelve years old.

can (is) are has

1. I ________ to get ready to leave.

   has begun begun began did begun

2. Both you and I ________ planning to go to the movies.

   were was is has

3. I'm tired of ________ in this chair.

   sitting setting satting has sat

4. Please ________ down and take a nap.

   lay lie lain lied

5. If you ________ to me, you wouldn't have gotten lost.

   listen are listening had listened was listening

6. The boys ________ out to the dock.

   swum had swimmed swam had swam

7. If you want me to, I ________ you a replacement.

   sent send have sent will send

8. Without his help, we ________ it.

   cannot have done will not had done

   could not did could not have done

9. I have just ________ War and Peace.

finishing read   finishing reading
finished read   finished reading

---

10. They should have ________ us.

told   have telled   tell   will tell

---

11. I sure ________ to win the prize money.

would hoped   are hoping   hope   will hope

---

12. I ________ to meet the man who wrote the book.

will liked   would like   met   would liken

---

13. All of us ________ what we want to eat.

will need deciding   will have to decide
will has to decide   will have decide

---

14. He tried ________ where the mouse was hiding.

founding   was found   looking   to find

---

15. I wish I ________ to lead the parade.

had been choosed   have chosen
had been chosen   had choosen

---

16. If he had had money, maybe he ________ .

will have succeeded   would have succeeded
could have succeeded   had succeeded

---

17. It's hard to believe that he ________ the piano before.

would never have played   had never play
has never played   never play

18. I had ________ what he looked like.

forget forgetted forgotten forgot

---

19. I am eating chocolate ice cream and she ________ vanilla.

am eating has ate is eating was ate

---

20. As John ________ the door, he dropped his book.

was opening open has opened opening

---

21. If you ________ , I would have been ready.

would call will call

had called will have called

---

22. I don't know when he ________ .

will go gone go has gone

---

23. I just finished ________ a letter to my aunt.

write written has written writing

---

24. She ________ in the Boston Marathon four times.

have ran has run has ran have run

---

25. She has not ________ for six months.

droven drive driven drove

---

26. The batter ________ out.

striked stricken struck strucked

Target Area 2: Morphemic Usage, Exercise 2

DIRECTIONS: The words in parentheses ( ) are all verbs. Fill in the blank with the correct form of the verb.

EXAMPLE: She (have) ___has___ twelve nieces and nephews.

1. The glass was (break) ________________ .
2. He (take) ________________ off his shirt because he was too hot.
3. Yesterday we (buy) ________________ a new set of tires.
4. Before we left, Mary (eat) ________________ her sandwich.
5. My husband (teach) ________________ me how to swim.
6. What have you (do) ________________ ?
7. She (tell) ________________ the police that she (lose) ________________ her wallet.
8. You should have (use) ________________ more soap.
9. Later this morning I (go) ________________ to the store for some milk.
10. The city (build) ________________ a new municipal office next year.
11. Even though we were (go) ________________ for six hours, we only (catch) ________________ two fish.
12. The baby (drink) ________________ the warm milk before she (go) ________________ to sleep.
13. Tomorrow you (know) ________________ whether you (pass) ________________ the test.
14. Last week four of us (hang) ________________ the wallpaper in the kitchen.

15. The tourists have (see) ______________________ many of the sights in the area.
16. The outfielder (catch) ______________________ three fly balls during the baseball game.
17. The dogs (run) ______________________ around the yard all afternoon.
18. My secretary (type) ______________________ the letters.
19. I (hear) ______________________ that you (get) ______________________ a new job a few months ago.
20. If you had (give) ______________________ the right directions, I would have (meet) ______________________ you on time.
21. He (fall) ______________________ when he (bend) ______________________ over to pick up a book.
22. After the bride (speak) ______________________ to the guests, she (throw) ______________________ the bouquet.
23. Last night a thief (break) ______________________ into the house and (steal) ______________________ our stereo equipment.
24. He (choose) ______________________ to (take) ______________________ the blue shirt instead of the red one.
25. I have (be) ______________________ awake since I (hear) ______________________ the alarm an hour ago.
26. The decision (is) ______________________ made before I (get) ______________________ there.

Target Area 2: Morphemic Usage, Exercise 3

DIRECTIONS: Fill in the blank with the correct word.

EXAMPLE: I went ___to___ the store.

1. I have five fingers ________ each hand.
2. She set the table ________ dinner.
3. I opened the bottle ________ a can opener.
4. We went out to dinner ________ there was nothing ________ eat in the house.
5. He cut the meat ________ a knife.
6. She weighed the vegetables ________ the scale.
7. I bought candy ________ the store.
8. I bought candy ________ the vendor.
9. I invited the men ________ my house.
10. ________ the game was over we went out ________ a drink.
11. We had a drink ________ water after jogging ________ the block.
12. Pete put his wallet ________ his pocket.
13. The bottle fell ________ the table.
14. This suit is different ________ mine.
15. He is the kind of person ________ would give you the shirt ________ his back.
16. Give me ________ apple, please.
17. Why don't you try ________ understand me.
18. Bill wants ________ buy a new puppy.
19. I received a birthday present ________ Aunt Mabel.

20. I think you should vote ________________ the Democratic candidate ________________ the Senate.
21. I can't decide ________________ type of lotion to buy.
22. ________________ I finish reading, I will go for a walk.
23. You can get a good meal at either the Mexican ________________ the Italian restaurant.
24. Could you direct me ________________ the nearest elevator?
25. The Chairman ________________ the Board is expected to come ________________ the meeting.
26. Look ________________ the word in the dictionary.
27. He doesn't know ________________ he will be able to come.
28. ________________ is the best time for me to call you?
29. The horse jumped ________________ the fence.
30. I will meet you ________________ three o'clock.

Target Area 2: Morphemic Usage, Exercise 4

DIRECTIONS: The following sentences are not correct. Rewrite each sentence so that it is correct.

EXAMPLE: Her is twelved years old yesterday.

She was twelve years old yesterday.

1. The pole vault record was broke yesterday. ______________________________

____

2. You and me should go there sometimes. ______________________________

____

3. The pipe had bursted into 3 parts. ______________________________

____

4. I'm glad that you brung the matter up today. ______________________________

____

5. I knowed it when he telled me about it. ______________________________

____

6. One of the puppy hasn't ate yet. ______________________________

____

7. The book fell back from off the chair. ______________________________

____

8. I couldn't find nobody whom would work of me. ______________________________

____

9. We hadn't hardly no time catching the bus. ______________________________

____

10. Either you come with me, nor me wont go. ____________________

____

11. If you had did what you was told, this wouldn't had happened. ____

____

____

12. Someone left their pen from the desk. ____________________

____

13. Her brother look a lot like she do. ____________________

____

14. Did he learn you how to do it? ____________________

____

15. When he hurting his arm, he stay in the hospital all night. ______

____

____

16. If you would have got the tickets sooner we would had had gooder seats. ____________________

____

17. After they seen us, they ask us to play a games for tennis. ______

____

18. Margarine are the best substitute of butter. ____________________

____

19. May I lend his pen off him for a minute? ____________________

____

20. Why don't you tried and be cooperation? ____________________

____

Target Area 2: Phrase Completions, Exercise 1

DIRECTIONS: Complete each phrase with a word or words so that the phrase makes sense. Use a different word for each phrase.

EXAMPLE: A dish of cereal

1. A drink of ______
2. A bunch of ______
3. A box of ______
4. A jar of ______
5. A stalk of ______
6. A loaf of ______
7. A dash of ______
8. A pack of ______
9. A tablespoon of ______
10. A bottle of ______
11. A lump of ______
12. A herd of ______
13. A vase of ______
14. A bag of ______
15. A pound of ______
16. A drop of ______
17. A flake of ______
18. A gallon of ______
19. A stick of ______
20. A tube of ______
21. A keg of ______
22. A carton of ______
23. A dab of ______

24. A cup of ________________

25. A slice of ________________

26. A pint of ________________

27. An ounce of ________________

28. A barrel of ________________

29. A bowl of ________________

30. A piece of ________________

31. A head of ________________

32. A pot of ________________

33. A pair of ________________

34. A load of ________________

35. A pitcher of ________________

36. A package of ________________

37. A teaspoonful of ________________

38. A bed of ________________

39. A drawer of ________________

40. A mug of ________________

41. A closet of ________________

42. A tray of ________________

43. A platter of ________________

44. A freezer of ________________

45. A crate of ________________

46. A bouquet of ________________

47. A pinch of ________________

48. A strip of ________________

49. An acre of ________________

50. A bit of ________________

51. A swarm of ________________

Target Area 2: Phrase Completions, Exercise 2

DIRECTIONS: Below are some familiar phrases that are incomplete. Complete each one with a word or words that will make the phrase complete and sensible.

EXAMPLE: As flat as a *pancake*

1. As blind as a ____________________
2. As cool as a ____________________
3. As neat as a ____________________
4. As fit as a ____________________
5. As stubborn as a ____________________
6. As slippery as an ____________________
7. As easy as ____________________
8. As smooth as ____________________
9. As pleased as ____________________
10. As American as ____________________
11. As fresh as a ____________________
12. As proud as a ____________________
13. As gentle as a ____________________
14. As snug as a ____________________ in a ____________
15. As busy as a ____________________
16. As clear as a ____________________
17. As thin as a ____________________
18. As dead as a ____________________
19. As clean as a ____________________
20. As innocent as a ____________________
21. As sweet as ____________________
22. As pretty as a ____________________

23. As sober as a ______________________________
24. As happy as a ______________________________
25. As hard as ______________________________
26. As slow as ______________________ in ____________
27. As quick as a ______________________________
28. As quiet as a ______________________________
29. As good as ______________________________
30. As playful as a ______________________________
31. As green as ______________________________
32. As white as a ______________________________
33. As smart as a ______________________________
34. As light as a ______________________________
35. As stiff as a ______________________________
36. As red as a ______________________________
37. As wise as an ______________________________
38. As big as a ______________________________
39. As flat as a ______________________________
40. As mad as a ______________________________
41. As straight as an ______________________________
42. As pale as a ______________________________
43. As sharp as a ______________________________
44. As sick as a ______________________________

Target Area 2: Phrase Completions, Exercise 3

DIRECTIONS: Below is a list of incomplete phrases. Finish each phrase with a word that will make sense. Use a different word or words in each phrase.

EXAMPLE: Try the *soup* ______________________________

1. Bend the ______________________________
2. Find the ______________________________
3. Turn the ______________________________
4. Use the ______________________________
5. Remind the ______________________________
6. Empty the ______________________________
7. Choose the ______________________________
8. Sail the ______________________________
9. Knit the ______________________________
10. Build the ______________________________
11. Connect the ______________________________
12. Boil the ______________________________
13. Operate the ______________________________
14. Rob the ______________________________
15. Refrigerate the ______________________________
16. Check the ______________________________
17. Dance the ______________________________
18. Frost the ______________________________
19. Pay the ______________________________
20. Sing the ______________________________
21. Open the ______________________________
22. Elect the ______________________________

23. Cook the ______
24. Stir the ______
25. Sharpen the ______
26. Clean the ______
27. Entertain the ______
28. Buy the ______
29. Ignore the ______
30. Meet the ______
31. Obey the ______
32. Add the ______
33. Practice the ______
34. Touch the ______
35. Discuss the ______
36. Carry the ______
37. Lick the ______
38. Rake the ______
39. Overlook the ______
40. Recognize the ______
41. Decorate the ______
42. Confess the ______
43. Give the ______
44. Begin the ______
45. Hear the ______
46. Weigh the ______
47. Wipe the ______
48. Fill the ______
49. Identify the ______
50. Interview the ______

Target Area 2: Phrase Completions, Exercise 4

DIRECTIONS: Below are some incomplete sentences. Begin each sentence with a word (or words) that will make sense. Use a different word in each sentence.

EXAMPLE: ___Pay___ the bill.

1. ______________ the bell.
2. ______________ the cigarette.
3. ______________ your teeth.
4. ______________ the pencil.
5. ______________ the song.
6. ______________ the kitchen floor.
7. ______________ your voice.
8. ______________ the envelope.
9. ______________ the film.
10. ______________ the daisy.
11. ______________ the beer.
12. ______________ the lightbulb.
13. ______________ the basket.
14. ______________ your birthday.
15. ______________ the gate.
16. ______________ the dog.
17. ______________ the coffee.
18. ______________ the furniture.
19. ______________ your nose.
20. ______________ the drawer.
21. ______________ the sink.
22. ______________ the child.

23. ________________________________ the casserole.
24. ________________________________ your money.
25. ________________________________ the weather.
26. ________________________________ the eggs.
27. ________________________________ the curtains.
28. ________________________________ the hem.
29. ________________________________ the lemon.
30. ________________________________ the tickets.
31. ________________________________ the fireplace.
32. ________________________________ the argument.
33. ________________________________ the language.
34. ________________________________ the reward.
35. ________________________________ your temper.
36. ________________________________ the experiment.
37. ________________________________ the wastebasket.
38. ________________________________ your elbow.
39. ________________________________ the opportunity.
40. ________________________________ the corn.
41. ________________________________ your neighbor.
42. ________________________________ the plant.
43. ________________________________ the model.
44. ________________________________ the performance.
45. ________________________________ the gum.
46. ________________________________ the magazine.
47. ________________________________ your diet.
48. ________________________________ your senator.
49. ________________________________ the army.
50. ________________________________ the field.

Target Area 2: Phrase Completions, Exercise 5

DIRECTIONS: The following sentences are incomplete. Each sentence has two or more blanks in it. Write a word (or words) in the blanks to make the sentence complete and sensible.

EXAMPLE: I like steak ________ but only if it is juicy ________ and rare ________ .

1. My brother took ________ bike and went for a ________ to the ________ .

2. The grocery store was ________ on Sunday so we bought some ________ and ________ for ________ .

3. Today the weather should be ________ and ________ with occasional ________ which will clear up by ________ .

4. I bought a new ________ at the ________ on ________ .

5. The ________ was ________ when I ________ it.

6. Please call ________ when you ________ or call ________ back ________ .

7. She ordered the ________ which was ________ and she had to ________ it.

8. Would you like to __________ today or would you like to __________ until __________ ?

---

9. The __________ present you __________ me was __________ and I'm so glad you __________ of __________ .

---

10. I want to __________ television because a special __________ is going to be __________ tonight.

---

11. I watched __________ last night and I slept __________ until __________ o'clock this morning.

---

12. He put on his __________ and then his __________ before he went to the __________ to see __________ .

---

13. The perfume smelled __________ when she __________ it on her __________ .

---

14. The woman is __________ a pot of __________ and baking some __________ for her __________ .

---

15. Before he __________ to bed, he __________ off his __________ and __________ his teeth with __________ .

16. The man tried on a ________________ pair of ________________ to see if they ________________ his ________________ sweater.

---

17. Boiling ________________ is ________________ to do.

---

18. I bought ________________ bags of ________________ at the ________________ .

---

19. She looks very ________________ today, but ________________ she looked even ________________ .

---

20. My ________________ plays the ________________ very ________________ .

---

21. I graduated from ________________ when I was ________________ .

---

22. ________________ picked us up at ________________ and ________________ us to see ________________ at the ________________ .

---

23. ________________ sister made ________________ sandwiches for Ed and ________________ to take to the ________________ .

24. He told me he ____________ the ____________ on your ____________ .

25. We had to ____________ because a ____________ had fallen across the ____________ .

26. Look at the ____________ woman with ____________ , ____________ hair and a ____________ dress sitting on the ____________ .

27. Suddenly a ____________ , ____________ dog raced across the ____________ yard and into the ____________ .

28. One ____________ , ____________ afternoon she went for a ____________ near the ____________ .

29. Mrs. ____________ gives ____________ lessons for ____________ an hour.

30. For sale: A ____________ in ____________ condition. Newly ____________ . It is ____________ in color and very ____________ . It's a real ____________ .

Target Area 2: Sentence Construction, Exercise 1

DIRECTIONS: Write one sentence that uses both words in it.

EXAMPLE: starts, acorn

An oak tree starts from an acorn.

1. reserve, theater ______________________________

____

2. after, interesting ______________________________

____

3. mystery, end ______________________________

____

4. apple, why ______________________________

____

5. distance, meet ______________________________

____

6. communicate, between ______________________________

____

7. exciting, introduction ______________________________

____

8. pass, horse ______________________________

____

9. bush, who ______________________________

____

10. car, yesterday ______________________________

11. very, appetite ______________________________

12. of, bear ______________________________

13. rainbow, notice ______________________________

14. note, tear ______________________________

15. tax, force ______________________________

16. forgive, whisper ______________________________

17. fork, use ______________________________

18. scarf, throw ______________________________

19. king, off ______________________________

20. anger, enough ______________________________

21. because, fever ______________________

____

22. thaw, this ______________________

____

23. gone, dictionary ______________________

____

24. out, brick ______________________

____

25. citizen, electing ______________________

____

26. near, peaches ______________________

____

27. rescue, without ______________________

____

28. floated, lady ______________________

____

29. arrange, play ______________________

____

30. climb, from ______________________

____

31. needle, short ______________________

____

32. ambition, neat ______________________________

____

33. great, any ______________________________

____

34. support, was ______________________________

____

35. still, keep ______________________________

____

36. traded, advantage ______________________________

____

37. found, pain ______________________________

____

38. rich, energy ______________________________

____

39. substitute, what ______________________________

____

40. camp, same ______________________________

____

Target Area 2: Sentence Construction, Exercise 2

DIRECTIONS: Write **one** sentence that uses all three words in it.

EXAMPLE: fix, wash, picnic *Wash your hands before you fix the food for the picnic.*

1. she, sell, talk ____________________

2. United States, know, life ____________________

3. close, group, this ____________________

4. deny, fights, seven ____________________

5. wrinkled, bought, sale ____________________

6. pound, aspirin, break ____________________

7. crust, bee, right ____________________

8. calendar, why, twenty ____________________

9. wood, trouble, money ____________________

10. clouds, when, lost ______________________________________

____

11. set, light, balcony ______________________________________

____

12. neglected, stand, young ______________________________________

____

13. wedding, hesitate, name ______________________________________

____

14. pollute, large, is ______________________________________

____

15. smooth, game, carry ______________________________________

____

16. ready, act, stretch ______________________________________

____

17. filling, appetite, safe ______________________________________

____

18. quickly, book, print ______________________________________

____

19. she, well, gave ______________________________________

____

20. summer, day, above ______________________________________

____

21. orange, into, six ______________________________

____

22. machine, magic, my ______________________________

____

23. super, listen, grand ______________________________

____

24. buffet, mouse, asparagus ______________________________

____

25. navy, vacation, leave ______________________________

____

26. really, known, today ______________________________

____

27. southern, nut, bring ______________________________

____

28. oars, figure, stay ______________________________

____

29. hurting, cause, office ______________________________

____

30. money, walk, answer ______________________________

____

31. baby, after, stones ______________________________

____

32. tired, lead, water ______________________________

____

33. sand, since, strain ______________________________

____

34. accent, from, nails ______________________________

____

35. trick, hoping, oven ______________________________

____

36. excited, weather, furry ___________________________

____

37. low, yellow, handkerchief _________________________

____

38. buttons, because, finished ________________________

____

39. seventeen, chin, then _____________________________

____

40. oil, gas, both ___________________________________

____

Target Area 2: Sentence Construction, Exercise 3

DIRECTIONS: Write a complete sentence that includes the given phrase.

EXAMPLE: once upon a time

Once upon a time I grew a beard.

1. in the town ______________________________

2. in a jiffy ______________________________

3. a large lake ______________________________

4. take a walk ______________________________

5. a warm day ______________________________

6. in a minute ______________________________

7. cream and sugar ______________________________

8. a red wagon ______________________________

9. have a milkshake ______________________________

10. running fast ______________________________
____

11. play ball ______________________________
____

12. afterwards ______________________________
____

13. a clean hanky ______________________________
____

14. on sale ______________________________
____

15. from the doctor ______________________________
____

16. heavier than most ______________________________
____

17. out to lunch ______________________________
____

18. a new liner ______________________________
____

19. never on time ______________________________
____

20. explained plainly ______________________________
____

21. putting in ______________________________

22. because it was ______________________________

23. just the right temperature ______________________________

24. stern but not harsh ______________________________

25. landed near the ______________________________

26. cancelled because of ______________________________

27. not very interesting ______________________________

28. can be hazardous ______________________________

29. trap sunlight ______________________________

30. too cheap ______________________________

31. heavy drinker ______________________________

32. joined before ______________________________

____

33. detailed maps ______________________________

____

34. high blood pressure ________________________

____

35. better than the rest _______________________

____

36. reached for ________________________________

____

37. usually depends on _________________________

____

38. a simple job _______________________________

____

39. rush hour traffic __________________________

____

40. not quite like _____________________________

____

Target Area 2: Paragraph Construction

DIRECTIONS: Write a **short** story using the words given below. Include at least one of the words in each sentence. The words do not have to be used in the same order as they are listed. Make the paragraph logical and complete. Underline the words as you use them. Use another sheet of paper for the paragraphs.

EXAMPLE: telephone, complete, busy, tonight, two, stay

I tried to call you tonight. Your telephone was busy for two hours. It was a complete waste of time for me to stay home and keep trying your number.

1. appetizing, onions, wine, garlic, linen, whispered, candlelight, sauce, afterwards, because

2. moving van, cartons, dusty, Illinois, exhausted, furniture, broken, without, 250, African violets

3. best seller, author, read, when, persuaded, paper, index, sold, love, review, often

4. educate, free, proof, college, realize, they, subjects, ability, student

5. of, on, into, Chevrolet, before, when, mileage, without, away, Ford

6. Swiss, years, call, Alps, lies, rich, our, trip, beautiful, this

7. cows, indicates, water, by, enemy, grass, exactly, around, summer, man

8. polls, vote, government, political, Congress, becomes, President, laws, taxes, campaign

---

9. airport, arriving, distance, required, health, United States, baggage, great, money, began

---

10. drink, smoke, touch, upon, tours, special, offices, noise, lines, approach

---

11. aphasia, hospital, rehabilitate, stroke, blood, write, language, first, speech, doctor

---

12. 20, friends, water, exercise, diet, bananas, money, fat, weight, lettuce

---

13. condominium, renovated, lease, security, rent, clubhouse, apartment, high, city, paint

---

14. call, May, travel, work, Mother's Day, many, brunch, rest, family, card

---

15. in, band, park, Sunday, free, stage, crowds, concert, no, chairs

---

16. fix, taxes, vote, speeches, register, open, promises, difference, ballots, Socialist

---

17. courses, discipline, pass, school, graduate, education, 18, fail, exams, because

---

18. return, the, money, when, without, caught, manager, mine, check, left

Target Area 3
LANGUAGE SEQUENCING

The exercises in Target Area Three are designed to aid the patient in redeveloping his ability to organize jumbled language stimuli. The recognition and organization of words when they are disguised or disarranged is a basic skill. Once he masters it, the patient can use this skill to cue himself on meanings without having to resort constantly to an analysis of language. The patient is not required to create an original response, but rather to sequence (or unscramble) language stimuli that have been disarranged purposely. This is a fundamental and widely accepted rehabilitation activity for the language-impaired patient.

The patient is asked to unscramble syllables, words, and sentences in individual exercises; he is also asked to identify smaller words contained in multisyllabic words, to sequence numbers, and to alphabetize. The exercises become increasingly difficult within each group, and the later exercises are particularly challenging. The Supplementary Materials section contains exercises that may be assigned in conjunction with this target area.

M.R.

Target Area 3: Scrambled Syllables, Exercise 1

DIRECTIONS: Match the syllable on the left with one on the right to form a word. Draw a line between the two correct syllables.

EXAMPLE:

with	keeper
book	draw
finger	nail

1. over	neath	4. rum	duce
under	break	stir	rup
house	room	val	tic
day	fold	pro	ue
blind	boat	plas	mage
store	head	bul	let
2. cheese	frog	5. sys	fer
waist	line	tack	tem
pocket	cake	wig	boo
bull	book	sug	le
barn	ever	pre	gle
for	yard	bam	gest
3. blos	dle	6. du	lapse
in	glar	su	ry
ser	vice	ju	der
o	stant	e	come
bur	pen	be	preme
sad	som	or	ty

7. en	ler
dan	mer
ant	cer
cor	ber
em	ter
sum	ner

8. ap	chor
ac	ing
act	plaud
a	mor
an	ble
ar	tion

9. pim	kle
bu	ble
sti	tle
bub	fle
lit	ple
wrin	gle

10. yel	el
vow	band
di	pare
pre	sil
hus	low
ton	ner

11. sham	miss
ze	let
an	noy
dis	lin
mus	ro
tab	poo

12. ig	fore
um	ture
pic	fire
be	pire
wel	nore
cross	fare

13. de	vite
re	tra
in	tress
for	gin
be	gion
ex	sire

14. bun	ly
Hen	ny
pan	by
ba	ry
la	dy
on	sy

15. rac	goon	19. box	boat
ma	roon	house	hound
car	phoon	grey	car
ty	poon	shoe	box
har	coon	snow	one
la	toon	some	flake
16. rum	pod	20. sin	turn
leg	jo	sau	gle
sol	end	tim	gan
tri	hale	or	to
ex	dier	au	ber
ban	mage	re	sage
17. sto	ple	21. ques	ta
stag	ry	quag	mire
stan	ble	quar	et
stum	dard	qui	tion
stee	ger	quo	ly
stu	pid	quick	rel
18. tem	cious	22. za	zag
gey	ser	zom	bra
bash	vice	zig	bie
gra	kle	zip	ny
ser	ful	ze	per
wrin	per	zir	con

23.	loz	chine	27.	hy	bout
	ma	sage		in	stall
	mas	cess		pro	file
	prin	er		e	ra
	riv	bal		vi	rus
	ver	enge		a	giene
24.	dis	row	28.	a	lect
	bor	turb		e	dore
	jas	fine		i	dor
	o	pal		o	cy
	rhu	per		u	ray
	de	barb		x	nit
25.	an	nor	29.	ex	age
	la	bor		un	sane
	par	sor		de	gain
	ho	kle		re	cuse
	liq	uor		in	fed
	cen	lor		im	fend
26.	shrink	gle	30.	Os	zel
	straw	ture		Lo	lix
	sprin	kle		Nan	is
	struc	berry		Ha	da
	stru	ing		Wan	car
	stran	del		Fe	cy

Target Area 3: Scrambled Syllables, Exercise 2

DIRECTIONS: Below are three-syllable words. Arrange the syllables in the correct order to form a word, and then write the word on the line.

EXAMPLE: ple ex am *example*

1. mal i an ______
2. vem ber No ______
3. gate nav i ______
4. der wil be ______
5. er pow ful ______
6. e el phant ______
7. hap ness pi ______
8. dar en cal ______
9. hood neigh bor ______
10. grate un ful ______
11. fy is sat ______
12. ous gen er ______
13. cue be bar ______
14. et book pock ______
15. ter is min ______
16. y ter pot ______
17. pus to oc ______
18. keep shop er ______
19. ci ac dent ______
20. ta to po ______
21. ven ad ture ______
22. tec tion pro ______

23. mem re ber ______________________________
24. ten lis ing ______________________________
25. mis per sion ______________________________
26. ty er prop ______________________________
27. age er av ______________________________
28. ous i cur ______________________________
29. trate con cen ______________________________
30. proof ter wa ______________________________
31. por tant im ______________________________
32. ment re tire ______________________________
33. i trop cal ______________________________
34. lo buf fa ______________________________
35. sid con er ______________________________
36. fish ly jel ______________________________
37. wall per pa ______________________________
38. man tic ro ______________________________
39. mum i max ______________________________
40. or tra ches ______________________________
41. ta quo tion ______________________________
42. le ath tic ______________________________
43. range ar ment ______________________________
44. ble sen si ______________________________
45. ter in rupt ______________________________
46. nar tive ra ______________________________
47. pen tine tur ______________________________
48. pre com hend ______________________________
49. cu cal late ______________________________
50. ar ette cig ______________________________

Target Area 3: Scrambled Syllables, Exercise 3

DIRECTIONS: Below are four-syllable words. Arrange the syllables in the correct order to form a word, and then write the word on the line.

1. a pre dic ment ____________________
2. or e vap ate ____________________
3. tics ma e math ____________________
4. o gra ge phy ____________________
5. in pen la su ____________________
6. ma ri te al ____________________
7. pen in dence de ____________________
8. ture ag ri cul ____________________
9. mo ter ther me ____________________
10. co al ho lic ____________________
11. com date ac mo ____________________
12. mi dor ry to ____________________
13. fac is sat tion ____________________
14. ble ta com for ____________________
15. tion si po dis ____________________
16. mer cy gen e ____________________
17. er lar pil cat ____________________
18. hel ter i cop ____________________
19. gre in di ent ____________________
20. mer A can i ____________________
21. ba ru ta ga ____________________
22. e cel bri ty ____________________
23. non a y mous ____________________

24. chu Mas sa setts ____________________
25. cin vac tion a ____________________
26. ment tise ver ad ____________________
27. nu al an ly ____________________
28. ni mag cent fi ____________________
29. ny cer e mo ____________________
30. mo co tive lo ____________________
31. to mo bile au ____________________
32. ti fer er liz ____________________
33. si sas nate as ____________________
34. sion ter mis in ____________________
35. ser ob tion va ____________________
36. der ing un stand ____________________
37. ra tion o dec ____________________
38. a tem ture per ____________________
39. on mel ter wa ____________________
40. al pro sion fes ____________________
41. a prob im ble ____________________
42. sip pi sis Mis ____________________
43. por trans tion ta ____________________
44. as ex ate per ____________________
45. men part de tal ____________________
46. ed ly doubt un ____________________
47. per a o tion ____________________
48. di com mo ty ____________________
49. lous i cu rid ____________________
50. cre ble di in ____________________

Target Area 3: Scrambled Words, Exercise 1

DIRECTIONS: If the following letters were unscrambled, they would form one of the four words given. Circle the word that is the correct answer.

EXAMPLE: Unscramble **l a b l**

labs able ball abel

1. Unscramble **f i l t**

   tilt flat lift trill

2. Unscramble **c r e s o**

   roses score prose scare

3. Unscramble **s t a t e**

   tests taste storm toast

4. Unscramble **l a o w l**

   lowly wallow allow lemon

5. Unscramble **f u l e t**

   felt left tulip flute

6. Unscramble **r o o c l**

   rocks locker coral color

7. Unscramble **d u i e g**

   ridge guile diets guide

8. Unscramble **r i s e n**

   snare north snored rinse

9. Unscramble **r r d o e**

   drove order doors rodeo

10. Unscramble **c h a t m**

match catch charm champ

---

11. Unscramble **m a r f e**

farms mare remain frame

---

12. Unscramble **w o r d s**

draws worms sword sorts

---

13. Unscramble **i n h k t**

thins kinky thing think

---

14. Unscramble **t h r o w**

worth thorn wrath rows

---

15. Unscramble **p s e u a**

apes pause paces pseudo

---

16. Unscramble **r h o b t**

throb berth robot brood

---

17. Unscramble **v e n e t**

tenet venus never event

---

18. Unscramble **i y s d a**

said daisy aides dyes

---

19. Unscramble **h c c o a**

coach cocoa choke chock

---

20. Unscramble **u b l i d**

blued double build label

---

21. Unscramble **t r a f e**

frame feared after freeze

22. Unscramble **c u r c o**

occur crush chorus crack

---

23. Unscramble **m u r h o**

huron humor rumor murky

---

24. Unscramble **h e r c a**

cheer share reach march

---

25. Unscramble **c k o h s**

chose husks shacks shock

---

26. Unscramble **c t h i k**

thick chick think chunk

---

27. Unscramble **n o a w g**

gone wagon gnaw gown

---

28. Unscramble **u t c o s**

stock cocker scout sketch

---

29. Unscramble **w r e o k r**

wrecker worker reword wrench

---

30. Unscramble **i n o g l e**

legion glowing olive legal

---

31. Unscramble **s e o r f t**

farthest trestle forest rotten

---

32. Unscramble **f e r f u s**

ruffle freaks useful suffer

---

33. Unscramble **r c e e l a**

clears cereal reels eclair

34. Unscramble **p s e r n o d**

person respond spores spoken

35. Unscramble **u t s e r e g**

gesture sturgeon greets greeting

36. Unscramble **l n e r y a**

rayon yearn learn nearly

37. Unscramble **m i s e p r s**

misery prison impress spire

38. Unscramble **p e c t c a**

accept pecan pacts catch

39. Unscramble **i y n r c g**

yearning curing racing crying

40. Unscramble **l l w w a o s**

llamas sallow willows swallow

41. Unscramble **l t a p e a**

plates palate talent paltry

42. Unscramble **t i g e m d**

midget edible magnet fidget

43. Unscramble **v e e l i b e**

veiled deliver evident believe

44. Unscramble **d s a n i l**

slain snails island denial

45. Unscramble **e c e r t s**

streak create strike secret

Target Area 3: Scrambled Words, Exercise 2

DIRECTIONS: Below are definitions with letters under them. Unscramble the letters and put them in order, making a word that fits the definition. The first letter of the correct word is already written.

EXAMPLE: something sweet to eat:

ynacd c a n d y

1. musical instrument with keys:

 oanpi p __ __ __ __

2. large farm usually for cattle:

 charn r __ __ __ __

3. long slithering animal:

 keans s __ __ __ __

4. someone who lives by himself:

 emirth h __ __ __ __ __

5. vegetable with a strong odor:

 inono o __ __ __ __

6. tall structure:

 trowe t __ __ __ __

7. the sound a duck makes:

 kaquc q __ __ __ __

8. spiny plant not needing much water:

 suctac c __ __ __ __ __

9. another name for billfold:

 lewalt w __ __ __ __ __

10. a breakfast drink:

 cijeu j __ __ __ __

11. be present somewhere:

    tadten a __ __ __ __ __

12. a direction:

    tronh n __ __ __ __

13. it makes dough rise:

    easty y __ __ __ __

14. not able to see:

    bildn b __ __ __ __

15. frosting on a cake:

    gnici i __ __ __ __

16. not clean:

    tridy d __ __ __ __

17. musical instrument:

    loiniv v __ __ __ __ __

18. stay on top of the water:

    atlof f __ __ __ __

19. big in size:

    garel l __ __ __ __

20. a small rat:

    seoum m __ __ __ __

21. place to live:

    meho h __ __ __

22. in addition to:

    trexa e __ __ __ __

23. eating tool:

    fenik k __ __ __ __

24. a sport:

    folg g __ __ __

25. rub very hard:

    crubs s __ __ __ __

26. how you get up a ladder:

    clibm c __ __ __ __

27. not old:

    gnuoy y __ __ __ __

28. a common flower:

    sadiy d __ __ __ __

29. place where you work:

    cefoif o __ __ __ __ __

30. what bees make:

    noyeh h __ __ __ __

31. a large fish:

    lehaw w __ __ __ __

32. a singing voice:

    treno t __ __ __ __

33. one who takes care of the sick:

    senur n __ __ __ __

34. type of bear:

    dapan p __ __ __ __

35. answer a question:

    plery r __ __ __ __

36. very young person:

    dilhc c __ __ __ __

37. book of maps:

    slata a __ __ __ __

38. built over water:

    debrig b __ __ __ __ __

Target Area 3: Scrambled Words, Exercise 3

DIRECTIONS: Unscramble the following words. Part of the new word is already shown. Fill in the missing letters with those given. Hint: Cross out the letters which have already been used in the answer.

EXAMPLE: Unscramble a s l s g s e g l a s s e s

1. Unscramble s t i l n e l i ___ ___ ___ n
2. Unscramble s t a m o l a l ___ ___ ___ ___
3. Unscramble s e x u c e e x ___ ___ ___ ___
4. Unscramble g a l i i n r o o r ___ g i ___ ___ l
5. Unscramble v s r e e e r r e ___ e ___ ___ e
6. Unscramble h e v s e n t s ___ ___ ___ ___ t h
7. Unscramble b e l t h i m t h ___ ___ ___ l e
8. Unscramble c e q h u n q u ___ ___ c ___
9. Unscramble r e c v i s e s ___ ___ ___ ___ c e
10. Unscramble y o m d e c c o ___ ___ ___ ___
11. Unscramble b e b l i r d d r ___ ___ ___ ___ e
12. Unscramble n o p i s o p ___ ___ ___ ___ n
13. Unscramble s s s e o t h h ___ ___ ___ ___ s s
14. Unscramble p i c s a l t p l ___ ___ ___ ___ c
15. Unscramble d c i h o r o r ___ ___ ___ ___
16. Unscramble w o e v l v ___ w ___ l
17. Unscramble e m y s t s s ___ s ___ ___ ___
18. Unscramble p c l u r e m ___ ___ ___ ___ p l e
19. Unscramble i t e m r e t t ___ r m ___ ___ e

20. Unscramble **m o r t s** ___ ___ ___ ___ m

21. Unscramble **p u z l e z** ___ ___ ___ z ___ ___

22. Unscramble **n o o n i** o ___ ___ o ___

23. Unscramble **e r i m d a** ___ d m ___ ___ ___

24. Unscramble **k n i g a t** ___ ___ ___ ___ ___ g

25. Unscramble **s u c s i s d** d ___ s ___ ___ s s

26. Unscramble **i s p u l m e** i ___ ___ u ___ ___ e

27. Unscramble **d a z i c o** z ___ ___ ___ ___ c

28. Unscramble **c l n i h f** ___ ___ ___ ___ c h

29. Unscramble **n c o o t t** ___ ___ t t ___ ___

30. Unscramble **t a u r e n** n ___ ___ ___ ___ e

31. Unscramble **l o d u s h** ___ ___ ___ ___ l d

32. Unscramble **s c i t t h** ___ t i t ___ ___

33. Unscramble **d i m a p r y** p y ___ ___ m ___ ___

34. Unscramble **t i l q y a u** ___ ___ ___ l ___ ___ y

35. Unscramble **c o y j e k** j ___ ___ ___ ___ y

36. Unscramble **t u g b e d** ___ ___ d g ___ ___

37. Unscramble **t e v a r i p** ___ ___ ___ v ___ t e

38. Unscramble **y e n t w t** ___ w ___ ___ ___ y

39. Unscramble **k a t m i s e** m ___ s t ___ ___ ___

40. Unscramble **w a r r o n** ___ ___ r r ___ ___

Target Area 3: Scrambled Words, Exercise 4

DIRECTIONS: Unscramble the words that belong to the category listed. Write the correct word in the blank next to the scrambled word. The first letter of the new word is capitalized.

EXAMPLE: **Animals**

g D o _dog_ _____

t a C _cat_ _____

s o u M e _mouse_ _____

1. **Colors**

d R e __________

c a l B k __________

w e l l o Y __________

W h e i t __________

u e l B __________

n i P k __________

r a n O e g __________

S e l r i v __________

o r w n B __________

y r a G __________

2. **Rooms in a house**

t n e i K c h ______

y i l F a m   m o o R ______

n e D ______

t r o m B a h o ______

s o l t e C ______

n i v g i L   o m o R ______

s a t n e B e m ______

r a n d y u L   o o m R ______

n n i i D g   m R o o ______

3. **Wild animals**

r a e B ______

n i o L ______

r i g e T ______

r a g o C u ______

C h a t e e h ______

l i G o r l a ______

r a b e Z ______

n a p E h e l t ______

f e r a f i G ______

r a o B ______

4. **European countries**

n E g n a l d ______

y a l I t ______

n a m G e r y ______

I e r l n a d ______

u m B e g l i ______

n a i p S ______

n a l d n i F ______

t r a i A u s ______

c e n F a r ______

t r o P u l a g ______

---

5. **Parts of the body**

m A r ______

p H i ______

w o b E l ______

g h i h T ______

s C e t h ______

s t i r W ______

c e N k ______

k e l A n ______

r e d o u l S h ______

e K e n ______

6. **Men's names**

t e b r R o ________________

a P u l ________________

s a m e J ________________

c a h R i d r ________________

n e H r y ________________

o e e G g r ________________

o h n J ________________

m i l i l a W ________________

g o D u ________________

l e a h c i M ________________

---

7. **Words beginning with sl—**

p e l S e ________________

d i l S e ________________

p l o S e ________________

h u l S s ________________

p r u l S ________________

S y y l l ________________

S n i g o p l ________________

v e r i l S ________________

n a g o l S ________________

d r e l e n S ________________

8. **Words beginning with thr—**

t e a r T h ______

f i t T y h r ______

n e T r o h ______

w T h r o ______

s h u r T h ______

l i h r l T ______

g h o u r h T ______

s t u r T h ______

t h o a T r ______

T e r e h ______

9. **Fruit**

h e C r y r ______

p a G e r ______

A p l e p ______

a c h e P ______

n o l e m r e t a W ______

a a a n n B ______

r b e y R a s r p ______

l b B r r e e y u ______

l a p P e p i n e ______

S y e r r r t w a b ______

10. **Cereals**

aiWheets ____________________

soierehC ____________________

ceRi rseiKips ____________________

noCr aleksF ____________________

maleOta ____________________

siinRa rBna ____________________

rheSdded etahW ____________________

rameC fo haeWt ____________________

cieR heCx ____________________

---

11. **Sports**

nigkSi ____________________

lofG ____________________

neTnis ____________________

lablaseB ____________________

mmiinwSg ____________________

nilrestWg ____________________

keycoH ____________________

notBinmad ____________________

olotFbla ____________________

12. **Holidays**

anitVelsen aDy ____________________

moMraeil yaD ____________________

utrFoh fo uJyl ____________________

eNw eraYs ____________________

shiatrmsC ____________________

asikTnghvnig ____________________

subomClu ayD ____________________

eteraVsn yDa ____________________

boraL ayD ____________________

thaFres aDy ____________________

---

13. **Women's names**

nasuS ____________________

yarM ____________________

olCra ____________________

caNny ____________________

noraSh ____________________

neJa ____________________

aniDe ____________________

raBraba ____________________

tanJe ____________________

aruLa ____________________

14. **Words ending in —ch**

e c h a R ______

t t a c h A ______

u c n L h ______

r A p o p c a h ______

t c h a M ______

A c r h ______

n u B h c ______

u c a L n h ______

t a c C h ______

a l B c h e ______

---

15. **Beverages**

d e n o m a L e ______

i M k l a h e k S ______

d I c e e a T ______

n a r O g e c i u J e ______

o e f e f C ______

i n e W ______

f o S t k r i D n ______

l i k M ______

r e B e ______

o C o a c ______

Target Area 3: Scrambled Sentences, Exercise 1

DIRECTIONS: Below are two columns of words. Pick words from column **a** and then from column **b** so that correct sentences are formed. Write the new sentences below the columns.

EXAMPLE:

a.	b.
I am	leave.
You will	hungry.

I am hungry.

You will leave.

a.	b.
The candle sticks	have a glass of wine.
I would like to	too long.
My pants are	are made of pewter.

1. ______________________
2. ______________________
3. ______________________

a.	b.
Ham and eggs	see him elected chairman.
We have lived in Troy	are good for breakfast.
I want to	for seven years.

4. ______________________
5. ______________________
6. ______________________

a.	b.
The cat is	sleeping by the chair.
I find your story	with his friends.
George is playing cards	hard to believe.

7. ______________________________
8. ______________________________
9. ______________________________

---

a.	b.
The Bicentennial was	in 1945.
World War II ended	in 1492.
Columbus discovered America	in 1976.

10. ______________________________
11. ______________________________
12. ______________________________

---

a.	b.
She needs to frost	the instructions.
He needs to wash	the chocolate cake.
He needs to read	the windows.

13. ______________________________
14. ______________________________
15. ______________________________

a.	b.
Put your money	in the dryer.
Put the clothes	in the bank.
Put the milk	in the refrigerator.

16. ______________________________
17. ______________________________
18. ______________________________

a.	b.
He went to the airport	to catch a plane.
He went to the drugstore	to get a suntan.
He went to the beach	to fill a prescription.

19. ______________________________
20. ______________________________
21. ______________________________

a.	b.
The river	vetoed the tax bill.
The president	had a strong current.
The little girl	dropped her candy.

22. ______________________________
23. ______________________________
24. ______________________________

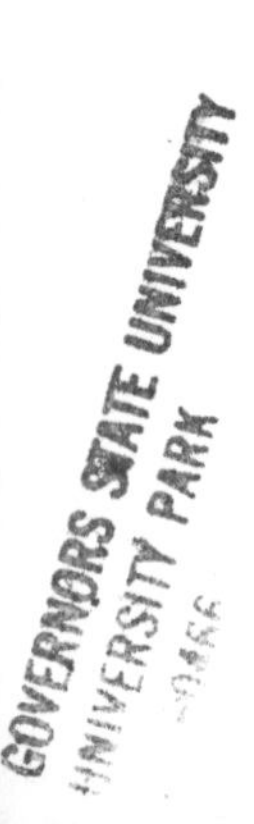

a.	b.
Please clean out	my apologies.
Please tell me	where Suite 200 is.
Please accept	the sink.

25. ______________________________

26. ______________________________

27. ______________________________

---

a.	b.
They have not	cocktail before dinner.
They are planning	to build a new house.
They didn't want a	paid their taxes yet.

28. ______________________________

29. ______________________________

30. ______________________________

---

a.	b.
I'll try to	anything to eat.
I haven't had	be there by seven.
I should buy	a new toaster soon.

31. ______________________________

32. ______________________________

33. ______________________________

Target Area 3: Scrambled Sentences, Exercise 2

DIRECTIONS: Continue as in previous exercise, using all three columns to put the sentences together.

a.	b.	c.
Water	are	plants.
Mr. Smith	the	sixty-five.
Coats	is	expensive.

1. ______________________
2. ______________________
3. ______________________

a.	b.	c.
Read	am	tired.
Please	be	me.
I	to	quiet.

4. ______________________
5. ______________________
6. ______________________

a.	b.	c.
Put	it	fast.
Jets	travel	sweet.
Sugar	is	down.

7. ______________________
8. ______________________
9. ______________________

a.	b.	c.
Roses	of	coffee.
Cup	the	stairs.
Up	are	red.

10. ____

11. ____

12. ____

---

a.	b.	c.
Smoke	Camel	bars.
Drink	Hershey	cigarettes.
Taste	Pepsi	Cola.

13. ____

14. ____

15. ____

---

a.	b.	c.
Mail	over	later.
Sink	or	swim.
Come	my	letter.

16. ____

17. ____

18. ____

a.	b.	c.
The zebra	that you came	a striped animal.
I'm glad	the horse	around the pasture.
He rode	is	to see me.

19. ________________________

20. ________________________

21. ________________________

---

a.	b.	c.
There's	don't have time	to see you.
I	is not the way	with me.
This	nothing wrong	to go.

22. ________________________

23. ________________________

24. ________________________

---

a.	b.	c.
May I borrow	they	of sugar?
Does it seem	a cup	will elect?
Whom do you think	like	he cares?

25. ________________________

26. ________________________

27. ________________________

a.	b.	c.
If we had	was full	we would.
The wastebasket	was over,	of garbage.
After the program	the chance,	I left.

28. ____________________
29. ____________________
30. ____________________

---

a.	b.	c.
Where do you	of pie	is this?
What kind	bus going	to eat?
When is the	want to go	to arrive?

31. ____________________
32. ____________________
33. ____________________

---

a.	b.	c.
The salad dressing	over the	tomato sauce.
Pour the syrup	contains	mayonnaise.
Add some onions	to the	pancakes.

34. ____________________
35. ____________________
36. ____________________

Target Area 3: Scrambled Sentences, Exercise 3

DIRECTIONS: Unscramble the words and put them in the correct order to form a sentence. Write the sentence. Hint: Cross out each word as you use it.

EXAMPLE: w~~a~~nt ~~I~~ co~~o~~kie ~~a~~ *I want a cookie*

1. sun today the is shining ______________________________

____

2. find can't my sweater I ______________________________

____

3. end street a this is dead ______________________________

____

4. time leave what we should? ______________________________

____

5. carefully the please bottle open ______________________________

____

6. was yesterday letter the mailed ______________________________

____

7. to peanuts like eat elephants ______________________________

____

8. for had pizza they dinner ______________________________

____

9. she where know went I don't ______________________________

____

10. you your what dog did name? ______________________________

____

11. remember we the books you where do put? ____________________

____

12. fire it the some logs needs on ____________________________

____

13. my chip cream favorite chocolate is ice ______________________

____

14. wearing the woman lovely a fur coat was _____________________

____

15. crackers bed should in never one eat ________________________

____

16. should to football what we game go time the? _________________

____

17. applesauce have dessert I want some for to ____________________

____

18. picked of peppers Piper peck Peter a pickled __________________

____

19. even suit this sale on it's though expensive is ________________

____

20. eggs coffee had breakfast scrambled juice I for and toast orange ___

____

____

21. Senate vetoed tax the the both the and House bill ________________

____

22. 200th States marked birthday 1976 the of the United ____________

____

23. so become went he lawyer to college could that a he ______________

____

24. eating cramps after soon go too get swimming might you if you

____

25. had tell me to hasn't she time news the ____________________

____

26. substitute in butter for can recipes margarine most you ___________

____

____

27. seven my quarts jam week of made strawberry neighbor last _______

____

28. schools parents would karate some like taught the in _____________

____

29. dress is next to lady the week in blue going the Italy ____________

____

30. Angeles the Olympics were 1984 Los summer in held in __________

____

31. calories milk 8 of 80 skim has ounces ______________________________

____

32. the thief money all cash the the stole register in ________________

____

33. entertainment watching of for is television a form many people ____

____

34. you succeed must confidence before have you can ______________

____

35. Tuesday the auto there is store sale at supply a ________________

____

36. patio on the mosquitos many are so there since inside go should we

____

____

37. an your before consult starting doctor on program exercise _______

____

38. inning were at fifth bases the the loaded bottom of the __________

____

____

39. played concert of symphony sonatas last a Beethoven the night ____

____

____

40. what don't send for I birthday to know her her ________________

____

Target Area 3: Words within Words

DIRECTIONS: Using only the letters in each word below, arrange the letters to form other, smaller words. Write down as many as you can find on another sheet of paper. You may use each letter only as many times as it appears in the given word.

EXAMPLE: weather *we, at, eat, rat, her, wet, wheat, heat, raw, war, tar, are, here, wear, hear, the*

1. telegraph
2. carnation
3. Washington
4. contribution
5. celebrate
6. telescope
7. millionaire
8. November
9. peculiarity
10. blackboard
11. alphabet
12. locomotive
13. relationship
14. schoolhouse
15. encyclopedia
16. understand
17. comfortable
18. automobile
19. kindergarten
20. headquarters
21. eliminate
22. panorama
23. timetable
24. vocabulary
25. bridesmaid
26. combination
27. literature
28. wardrobe
29. anticipated
30. watermelon

Target Area 3: Numerical Sequencing, Exercise 1

DIRECTIONS: Rearrange the following numbers in order from the **smallest to the largest** and write them on the lines.

EXAMPLE:

17	2	2	14
21	6	6	17
14	12	12	21

a. 92 ______
36 ______
29 ______
47 ______
63 ______
18 ______

b. 63 ______
39 ______
78 ______
47 ______
79 ______
24 ______

c. 97 ______
68 ______
27 ______
45 ______
58 ______
17 ______

d. 23 ______
14 ______
63 ______
45 ______
29 ______
16 ______

e. 127 ______
172 ______
146 ______
122 ______
176 ______
145 ______

f. 163 ______
147 ______
132 ______
161 ______
153 ______
140 ______

g. 133 ______
164 ______
122 ______
145 ______
178 ______
196 ______

h. 127 ______
194 ______
183 ______
169 ______
144 ______
126 ______

i. 329 ______
165 ______
252 ______
497 ______
763 ______
641 ______

j.	k.	l.
647	646	542
392	464	561
864	297	547
397	342	536
673	269	529
542	199	575

m.	n.	o.
3,605	564	5,140
2,140	1,947	2,397
762	6,333	6,420
4,925	1,651	2,381
6,274	3,692	8,291
1,473	7,490	5,450
430	3,249	7,365
5,645	7,489	9,291

p.	q.	r.
9,641	9,652	36,255
2,346	7,453	794
7,930	2,599	6,565
5,624	1,642	82,147
3,955	5,546	845
6,430	6,049	62,395
9,285	5,460	8,549
4,547	7,925	73,501

s.		t.	
82,359	______	49,864	______
6,254	______	26,543	______
3,981	______	465	______
70,239	______	3,925	______
8,925	______	16,933	______
67,488	______	259	______
72,945	______	89,285	______
35,497	______	3,927	______
9,254	______	5,834	______
864	______	65,243	______
90,487	______	725	______
453	______	8,639	______
7,730	______	73,501	______

Target Area 3: Numerical Sequencing, Exercise 2

DIRECTIONS: Rearrange the following numbers in order, from the **largest to smallest,** and write them on the lines.

EXAMPLE:

17	21	2	12
21	17	6	6
14	14	12	2

a.		b.		c.	
36	______	93	______	67	______
10	______	60	______	40	______
75	______	88	______	62	______
32	______	17	______	37	______
54	______	36	______	92	______
68	______	54	______	46	______

d.		e.		f.	
32	______	172	______	136	______
41	______	127	______	174	______
47	______	164	______	123	______
54	______	133	______	116	______
92	______	167	______	135	______
61	______	154	______	104	______

g.		h.		i.	
183	______	173	______	923	______
146	______	149	______	561	______
122	______	138	______	252	______
154	______	196	______	146	______
187	______	144	______	794	______
169	______	172	______	367	______

j.		k.		l.	
	746 ______		646 ______		245 ______
	293 ______		464 ______		264 ______
	468 ______		792 ______		247 ______
	245 ______		991 ______		157 ______
	793 ______		243 ______		263 ______
	379 ______		296 ______		292 ______

m.		n.		o.	
	5,063 ______		464 ______		4,150 ______
	4,410 ______		7,491 ______		7,932 ______
	267 ______		3,336 ______		4,206 ______
	5,294 ______		1,561 ______		1,832 ______
	4,726 ______		2,963 ______		1,928 ______
	3,741 ______		3,974 ______		5,054 ______
	340 ______		7,942 ______		5,637 ______
	5,465 ______		9,857 ______		1,929 ______

p.		q.		r.	
	1,469 ______		2,569 ______		55,263 ______
	6,432 ______		3,547 ______		497 ______
	3,970 ______		9,952 ______		5,654 ______
	4,264 ______		2,461 ______		74,128 ______
	5,559 ______		6,455 ______		548 ______
	3,034 ______		9,406 ______		59,326 ______
	5,829 ______		6,045 ______		9,458 ______
	7,454 ______		5,297 ______		72 ______

s. 95,328 ____________
4,526 ____________
1,893 ____________
93,207 ____________
5,298 ____________
88,476 ____________
54,927 ____________
79,453 ____________
4,524 ____________
468 ____________
78,409 ____________
354 ____________
45,083 ____________

t. 46,894 ____________
34,652 ____________
564 ____________
5,293 ____________
33,961 ____________
952 ____________
58,298 ____________
9,293 ____________
4,385 ____________
34,256 ____________
527 ____________
9,368 ____________
10,537 ____________

Target Area 3: Numerical Sequencing, Exercise 3

DIRECTIONS: Draw a line from the numeral on the left to the equivalent word on the right.

EXAMPLE:

9	seventeen
17	twelve
12	nine
4	four

a.

1,003	one thousand one hundred thirty
1,013	one thousand three hundred ten
1,130	one thousand three
1,310	one thousand thirteen

---

b.

640	four hundred sixty
460	six hundred four
604	six hundred forty
464	four hundred sixty-four

---

c.

2,735	two thousand seven hundred thirty-five
2,035	two thousand thirty-five
2,075	two thousand seventy-five
2,705	two thousand seven hundred five

---

d.

600,000	six hundred sixty thousand
60,000	sixty thousand
606,000	six hundred six thousand
6,000	six hundred thousand
660,000	six thousand

e.	1,000	ten thousand
	100,000	one thousand
	10,000	one hundred thousand
	101,000	one hundred one thousand
f.	7,727	seven thousand seven hundred twenty-seven
	7,272	seven thousand two hundred seventy-two
	2,772	two thousand two hundred seventy-seven
	2,277	two thousand seven hundred seventy-two
g.	900,001	nine hundred thousand nine hundred one
	909,001	ninety thousand one
	90,001	nine hundred nine thousand one
	900,901	nine hundred thousand one
h.	8,646	eight thousand eight hundred sixty-four
	8,464	eight thousand four hundred sixty-four
	8,864	eight thousand six hundred forty-six
	8,846	eight thousand eight hundred forty-six
i.	55,505	fifty-five thousand five hundred fifty-five
	50,550	fifty thousand fifty-five
	50,055	fifty thousand five hundred fifty
	55,555	fifty-five thousand five hundred five
j.	2,222	two thousand two hundred two
	2,022	two thousand twenty-two
	2,202	two thousand two hundred twenty
	2,220	two thousand two hundred twenty-two

k.	333	thirty-three thousand three hundred thirty-three
	333,333	three hundred thirty-three thousand three hundred thirty-three
	33,333	three thousand three hundred thirty-three
	3,333	three hundred thirty-three
l.	17,717	seventy-one hundred seventeen
	71,117	seventeen hundred seventeen
	1,717	seventy-one thousand one hundred seventeen
	7,117	seventeen thousand seven hundred seventeen
m.	48,480	forty-eight hundred eighty
	4,880	four hundred forty-eight thousand eight hundred forty-four
	448,844	four thousand four hundred eighty
	4,480	forty-eight thousand four hundred eighty
n.	80,008	eight hundred eight
	8,008	eighty-eight hundred eight
	8,808	eighty hundred eight
	808	eighty thousand eight
o.	2,002,002	two million two hundred two thousand twenty
	2,202,020	two million two hundred two thousand two
	2,202,002	two million two thousand two
	2,002,020	two million two thousand twenty
p.	1,010,000	one million one hundred
	101,000,000	one million one hundred thousand
	1,100,000	one hundred one million
	1,000,100	one million ten thousand

q.	4,321	forty-three thousand twenty-one
	40,321	forty-three thousand two hundred one
	43,021	forty thousand three hundred twenty-one
	43,201	forty-three hundred twenty-one
r.	111,111	eleven hundred eleven
	1,111,111	one hundred eleven thousand one hundred eleven
	1,111	one million one hundred eleven thousand one hundred eleven
	11,111	eleven thousand one hundred eleven
s.	949,494	nine hundred forty-nine thousand four hundred ninety-four
	94,949	four hundred ninety-four thousand nine hundred forty-nine
	494,949	forty-nine thousand four hundred ninety-four
	49,494	ninety-four thousand nine hundred forty-nine
t.	6,016	six thousand sixty-six
	6,066	six thousand sixty
	6,060	six thousand sixteen
	6,116	sixty-one hundred sixteen

Target Area 3: Numerical Sequencing, Exercise 4

DIRECTIONS: Write out the numbers below in words.

EXAMPLE: 284 *two hundred eighty-four*

a. 387 ______

b. 946 ______

c. 101 ______

d. 6,208 ______

e. 1,367 ______

f. 3,008 ______

g. 2,130 ______

h. 16,300 ______

i. 25,002 ______

j. 88,888 ______

k. 655-1/2 ______________________________

____

l. 98,926 ______________________________

____

m. 1,000,001 ______________________________

____

n. 606,280 ______________________________

____

o. 1,444,444 ______________________________

____

a. $1.25 ______________________________

____

b. $13.50 ______________________________

____

c. $101.00 ______________________________

____

d. $10.04 ______________________________

____

e. $97.52 ______________________________

____

f. $132.47 ______________________________

____

g. $87.84 ____________________

____

h. $50.05 ____________________

____

i. $103.63 ____________________

____

j. $1,240.00 ____________________

____

k. $640.06 ____________________

____

l. $7,132.65 ____________________

____

m. $3,003.03 ____________________

____

n. $1,000,000.05 ____________________

____

o. $999,999.99 ____________________

____

Target Area 3: Alphabetizing, Exercise 1

DIRECTIONS: Write the alphabet below.

____

____

Rearrange the words in each of the lists below so that they are in **alphabetical order.**

EXAMPLE:

hair ____ apple

apple ____ hair

money ____ money

1. bagel ____
   lamp ____
   roast ____
   corn ____
   train ____
   oasis ____

2. yarn ____
   popcorn ____
   kernel ____
   opinion ____
   desert ____
   needle ____

3. horn ____
   listen ____
   whale ____
   seat ____
   key ____
   boat ____

4. bean ____
   alarm ____
   garage ____
   dump ____
   orange ____
   kite ____

5. numbers ________
   handle ________
   above ________
   finger ________
   jelly ________
   raisin ________

6. open ________
   indoors ________
   alarm ________
   under ________
   penguin ________
   yard ________

7. snake ________
   allow ________
   cover ________
   engine ________
   split ________
   active ________
   cactus ________
   bush ________

8. out ________
   paw ________
   drawn ________
   hound ________
   comfort ________
   multiply ________
   remain ________
   elevate ________

9. bakery ________
   absent ________
   member ________
   product ________
   vein ________
   friend ________
   yearn ________
   shriek ________

10. lane ________
    stolen ________
    neat ________
    kiss ________
    miss ________
    parsley ________
    oven ________
    jaws ________

11. zeal ______
worth ______
x-ray ______
quiet ______
yet ______
violin ______
risk ______
loop ______

12. copy ______
beer ______
axe ______
grab ______
fox ______
dread ______
expect ______
hot ______

13. husk ______
drift ______
concern ______
nearly ______
junior ______
spicy ______
python ______
involve ______

14. jade ______
pleasant ______
litter ______
thicket ______
unwilling ______
inhale ______
gong ______
resist ______

15. truce ______
profound ______
found ______
drapes ______
berth ______
raise ______
twitch ______
cereal ______

16. dugout ______
wasp ______
beacon ______
alto ______
wrist ______
ramrod ______
heave ______
tact ______

17. table ______
ace ______
fawn ______
range ______
knight ______
tavern ______
quarter ______
oblige ______

18. muscle ______
hedge ______
orphan ______
crystal ______
buffet ______
replace ______
program ______
shrink ______

19. tax ______
delicious ______
curb ______
pepper ______
tackle ______
ransom ______
cotton ______
last ______

20. hoarse ______
scout ______
tender ______
comedy ______
shady ______
apron ______
drama ______
repeat ______

21. principal ______
improvise ______
violets ______
tuition ______
technical ______
circulate ______
muscular ______
quite ______

22. shrubbery ______
rummage ______
transistor ______
vibrate ______
utilize ______
recover ______
vacation ______
yardstick ______

Target Area 3: Alphabetizing, Exercise 2

DIRECTIONS: Rearrange the words in each of the lists below so that they are in alphabetical order.

1. beanstalk ______	2. ruin ______
beast ______	rumor ______
beef ______	rein ______
bee ______	read ______
bear ______	rear ______
beer ______	rare ______
3. learn ______	4. opposite ______
last ______	open ______
lame ______	opinion ______
least ______	Ophelia ______
lamp ______	only ______
late ______	on ______
5. catch ______	6. music ______
caught ______	mirror ______
cent ______	more ______
cinder ______	most ______
cast ______	make ______
camp ______	meant ______

7. irk ________
in ________
is ________
if ________
ink ________
it ________

8. expect ________
expert ________
extinct ________
x-ray ________
extra ________
exert ________

9. nick ________
nil ________
nigh ________
nitrogen ________
nice ________
nifty ________

10. hymn ________
hydrogen ________
hydrant ________
hyphen ________
hypnotist ________
hyperbole ________

11. tractor ________
track ________
trachea ________
tract ________
traction ________
trace ________

12. physical ________
psychic ________
physics ________
python ________
phrase ________
phylum ________

13. accident ________
academy ________
ache ________
auto ________
actor ________
air ________

14. zinc ________
zany ________
zodiac ________
zero ________
zigzag ________
zeal ________

15. knead ______________________
knuckle ______________________
knife ______________________
koala ______________________
knob ______________________
knot ______________________

16. dandruff ______________________
dilemma ______________________
descend ______________________
druggist ______________________
dugout ______________________
dagger ______________________

17. squalor ______________________
squabble ______________________
squander ______________________
squad ______________________
square ______________________
squash ______________________

18. veteran ______________________
vertigo ______________________
vessel ______________________
venerate ______________________
velvet ______________________
vex ______________________

19. gas ______________________
gasp ______________________
gaseous ______________________
gash ______________________
gastric ______________________
gassy ______________________

20. rule ______________________
yogurt ______________________
yucca ______________________
yummy ______________________
Yukon ______________________
yoyo ______________________

21. fossil ______________________
fiddle ______________________
final ______________________
fertile ______________________
fiber ______________________
fizzle ______________________

22. path ______________________
pat ______________________
patch ______________________
patio ______________________
pattern ______________________
patter ______________________

Target Area 4

FOLLOWING WRITTEN DIRECTIVES

The dyslexic patient often has difficulty comprehending factual or complex written material, and may complain of the amount of time he needs to absorb what, in his pre-morbid state, he understood readily. The patient who had once enjoyed reading may now find it a time-consuming chore. In Target Area Four the patient is directed to attend to detailed written instructions, and consequently to focus on the meaning of the written word. The recovery of this ability to process detailed material is vital to the patient who wishes to employ his reading skills for recreational or occupational purposes.

Several exercises in this target area ask the patient to indicate his comprehension by giving simple responses such as checking, circling, or crossing out words. Other exercises require him to follow a series of detailed directions in answering each question. The exercises with numbers, in line with the concerns of this section, concentrate on developing the patient's ability to carefully consider the given instructions—and carry them through—rather than stress actual computation. Finally, several exercises in the Supplementary Materials section coordinate well with this target area.

M.R.

Target Area 4: Comprehension of Instructions

DIRECTIONS: Each question has different instructions. Answer each question by doing **exactly as the instructions direct.**

EXAMPLE: Add an **s** to every word.

apple s   cat s   house s   bottle s

1. Underline all the words ending in **ch**.

   peach   charm   watch   hatchet   wash

---

2. Circle the vowel following the two letters that are the same.

   bigger   cattle   kitten   appear   saddest

---

3. Put a triangle over all of the words with six letters.

   horns   hatchet   opener   listen   musket

---

4. Circle the second **d** below.

   Underline all **o**'s.

   Put a box around the third **y**.

   Place a dot under all of the **s**'s.

   r a p d s b o e y c d y o r s q p t r o t y l p d

---

5. Circle the letter that follows each **s** in the words below.

   super   system   assistant   shadiest   sisters

---

6. If a cat has whiskers, cross out the third word. If cabbage has pods, cross out the last word. If cabbage does **not** have pods, go on to the next question.

   haunt   limit   exciting   water   difficult

---

7. Put a check in front of all of the words that rhyme with **sap**.

   strap   sag   strip   lap   trap

8. Circle the words that begin with the same letter that **cat** begins with.

   certain absolutely positive captivate endearing

---

9. Add the letters **ing** to each word beginning with the letters **sh**.

   accept shorten sharpen cheapen

---

10. Underline the words that refer to a person in the sentence below.

    The boy in the green sweater was the one to whom I delivered candy.

---

11. Cross out the last two letters of each word.

    company rooster antique Atlantic executive

---

12. Check the words meaning things that belong in the kitchen.

    utensils mayonnaise income banister faucet

---

13. Put a triangle above the word that does not belong.

    apples radishes cherries lettuce tomatoes

---

14. Circle all of the **a**'s, **r**'s, and **e**'s in each of the following words:

    butter exciting mirror monument career

---

15. Put a box around the words with less than six letters.

    hatchet alone carpenter sincere opal

---

16. If horses fly, cross out the last word. If they don't, skip this question.

    listening walking flying running singing

---

17. Put a dot over any words that rhyme with **pour**.

    tour for tore sour our

18. Put marks in front of the words that begin with the same letter as **behind** ends with.

island dent iron dig garage

---

19. Add the letters **ment** to the words that do **not** end in **e**.

attain content excite advise adorn

---

20. Underline any word that tells **when**.

I went to the store on Tuesday for some bread.

---

21. Mark an **x** underneath the last letter of each color.

red blue plant cherry white

---

22. Circle any word that belongs with a fork.

kitchen sand knife baby spoon

---

23. Put a line over the words that begin with **st**.

same strain fast investment sty

---

24. Make a cross over the consonants in the following words.

team over ace hoop horizon

---

25. Put a circle over the words that have eight letters.

concern turbulent possible response argument

---

26. Put a square above all the **b**'s.

Circle any of the letters below that are in the word **cry**.

Cross out all of the letters that come before **f** in the alphabet.

Put a triangle under the second **b** and the first **m**.

r y p s b y c d g m s j o y c b b l o m n q i b c r

---

27. Underline the letters that appear before each **t** in the following words.

entertain exactly apartment intention artist

28. If baby sheep are called lambs do **not** cross out any words. If they are **not** called lambs, cross out the second word.

box egg yellow curt tame

---

29. Cross out the words that do not rhyme with **lane**.

sane pain lain fine loin

---

30. Write **yes** over the words that end with the same letter that **dog** begins with.

desire dead opened food dig

---

31. Draw a line through the last syllable of the following words.

appointment lotion following open vacation

---

32. Underline the words that tell **how** in the following sentence.

With a quick tug on the end of the rope, he was able to land the fish in the boat.

---

33. In the following words, circle all the letters that appear in **act.**

exactly catcher tactile actually pointed

---

34. Put a dot in front of the words that are longer than the word **short**.

tall ankle flower bowling oil

---

35. Add the letter **m** to the beginning of each word and write the new word above the original word.

any ore ice other eat

---

36. Cross out the shortest word and circle the longest word.

rooster expect alone oats master

---

37. Put a check over the animal, a circle in front of the color, a cross through the fruit, and a square around the vegetable.

Indian ox squash yellow prune

38. If May comes after June, circle the third word. If it does not, draw a line through the first word.

ring box mug plate phone

---

39. Write the opposite of each word above the original word.

down falling yes under top

---

40. Above the sport mark a √. Cross out the number and circle the jewelry. Put a line through the liquid and put a square around the musical instrument.

bracelet hockey violin seven milk

---

41. Cross out the word below that means the same as **magnify.**

decrease enlarge copy repeat

---

42. Draw arrows pointing to the words which are also words if they are spelled backwards.

deer pool plan drawer slit

---

43. Put numbers over each word so that the longest word is number **1,** the shortest word is number **2,** and the word with the most vowels is number **3.**

excited late accident avenue

---

44. Write **no** above the words that are cities. Write **yes** below the words that are not.

Dallas Dynasty Chicago Hotel Jamaica

---

45. Count the number of **i**'s in the sentence below and write that number above the fourth word.

"Be kind to animals" is good advice.

Target Area 4: Specific Directions

DIRECTIONS: For these exercises you must follow **specific directions**. You will need another sheet of paper. Do **exactly** as the directions indicate for each question, as each question has different directions.

a.

1. You will need a blank sheet of paper.
2. Make a small circle in the center of the sheet.
3. Write the number **3** in the center of the circle.
4. Write your name in the upper left corner of the paper.
5. Write the date in the lower right corner of the paper.
6. Just below the circle, write the word **pony**.
7. Along the upper right edge of the paper, write the first five letters of the alphabet.
8. Halfway between the circle and the bottom of the page, write a sentence describing the weather.
9. In the upper half of the page, write three words describing winter.
10. Write the numbers from **1** to **10** backwards down the left side of the page.
11. Fold the entire page in half the long way.

b.

1. Fold a piece of paper in half, then unfold it again.
2. Draw a box anywhere on the bottom half of the sheet of paper.
3. To the right of the box, write the name of an animal.
4. Write your shoe size inside the box.
5. Draw a straight line down from the bottom edge of the box to the bottom of the page.
6. Divide this line in half with a short horizontal line.
7. On the other half of the folded sheet, draw three circles in three different sizes.
8. Put a check mark above the smallest circle and a cross below the largest circle.
9. Turn the paper over.
10. Somewhere on that side of the paper, write the name of the place where you were born.
11. Underline three times the name of the state in which you were born.
12. Above that, print the name of the place where you now live.
13. Circle the name of the city in which you now live.

c. Follow the directions below the list of words, **exactly** as indicated.

envelope	antelope	green
tan	hunt	turkey
purple	white	broccoli
beet	kangaroo	corn
bear	talent	violet
igloo	brown	leopard
tape	beaver	street
pea	ashtray	turnip

1. Underline all the animals once.
2. Circle all words with two or more **e**'s in them.
3. Underline all the vegetables twice.
4. Put a cross through all the words that either begin or end with the letter **t**.
5. Put a $\surd$ in front of each color.
6. Put a star next to the words that are more than six letters long.

d.

George	Anna	New York
Alabama	Boston	David
Germany	Rockefeller	Atlanta
Oregon	Samuel	Alaska
Jane	Ohio	Sacramento
Bob	Dorothy	Hannah
Florida	river	Arizona
Africa	Delaware	Long Island
Allegheny	Colorado	Honolulu

1. Put a line through all the men's names.
2. Underline once all the women's names.
3. Circle the names of states in the United States.
4. Put two lines under all states east of the Mississippi River.
5. Put a check next to all the words beginning and ending with the same letter.
6. Copy the names of the state capitals in the space below.

e. Follow the directions below exactly.

1. Print the word **hamburger** on the line below.

____

2. Switch the places of the **a** and the **e** in the word. Now rewrite the word.

____

3. Switch the places of the **h** and the **m**. Now rewrite the word.

____

4. Cross out the **b**, then replace the **u** with a **t**. Now rewrite the word.

____

5. Replace the first **r** with an **l**, and the second **r** with an **f**. Rewrite the word.

____

6. Change the sixth letter to an **o**. Now rewrite the word.

____

7. Change the **h** to the same letter as the second to the last letter. Rewrite the word.

____

8. The word should now be the name of a food made from hamburger. Write it.

____

f. Follow the directions below exactly.

1. Print the word **microwave** on the line below.

   ____

2. Switch the places of the **w** and the **a** in the word. Now rewrite the word.

   ____

3. Switch the places of the **i** and the **o.** Now write the word.

   ____

4. Change the first letter to an **a,** and change the next to the last letter to a **c.** Rewrite the word.

   ____

5. Change the second and third letters to **p**'s. Rewrite the word.

   ____

6. Cross out the fourth letter and change it to an **l.** Change the seventh letter to an **n.** The letters should spell the category a microwave oven belongs to. Rewrite the new word.

   ____

g. Follow the directions below exactly.

1. Print the word **apartment** on the line below.

____

2. In the word you just printed, change the first **a** to a **c,** and the second **a** to an **n.** Cross out both **t**'s. Rewrite the word with the new letters.

____

3. In the word on the line above, cross out the **e.** Add an **i** on both sides of the second **n.** Rewrite the new word.

____

4. Replace the **p** with an **o.** Place another **o** between the **r** and the **m.** Rewrite the new word.

____

5. Add **u** and **m** to the end of the word. Cross out the **r** and put a **d** in its place. Rewrite the new word.

____

6. The letters should spell a word that describes what some apartments become. Write the new word on the line below.

____

h. Follow the directions below exactly.

Column A	Column B	Column C
organ	oldest	loaded
typist	hydrant	scared
after	jacket	monument
lost	tuba	calendar
eraser	barber	voted
dollar	varnish	twenty
harness	acrobat	penguin
lace	meatballs	rhythm

1. In Column C, put a box around the number that is listed.
2. Put a star after the third word in Column A.
3. In Column B, underline the two words that name people's jobs.
4. Put quotes around a type of money in Column A.
5. In the same column, put a box around a piece of equipment used with a horse.
6. Place a star next to the third to last word in the second column.
7. Star the word meaning **frightened.**
8. In Column B, put in quotes the name of a musical instrument.
9. Put the bird in Column C in quotes.
10. Underline **monument** where it appears above.
11. In which column is the word meaning the opposite of **found**?

    ____

12. In which column does a kind of food appear?

    ____________________ What is it? ____________________

i. Follow all the directions below exactly.

Column 1	Column 2	Column 3
lemon	green	iceberg
allow	corner	leather
wedge	itch	wheels
happy	order	hard
under	scold	whisper
toad	wasp	radio
aspirin	tongue	bought
plug	ordinary	sink

1. In the middle column, cross out the third word.
2. In Column 1, circle the word meaning **glad**.
3. Circle the second to last word in the second column.
4. Put a box around the word in Column 3 meaning a material often used for shoes.
5. Check the word in the first column meaning an **amphibian.**
6. In Column 3, check the word meaning the opposite of **soft**.
7. Cross out the words in Column 1 that begin with the first letter of the alphabet.
8. Make a check beside the word **corner**.
9. Put a box around a type of medicine in Column 1.
10. Cross out the coldest thing in Column 3.
11. In which column is the word **plug**? ____________________
12. In which column is the word meaning an insect?

____

Target Area 4: Numerical Reasoning, Exercise 1

DIRECTIONS: Follow the directions given for each question.

EXAMPLE: Circle the number under 5.

(2) 7 8 14

1. Circle the correct answer to each question.

a. Which number is closest to 78?

62 87 46 93

---

b. Which number is closest to 16?

25 10 24 12

---

c. Which number is closest to 52?

48 57 25 50

---

d. Which number is closest to 87?

91 76 80 85

---

e. Which number is closest to 240?

265 221 260 253

---

f. Which number is closest to 163?

100 150 125 253

---

g. Which number is closest to 1,000?

842 623 845 450

2. Answer the following questions on the line provided.

   a. 6 4 2 5 5 4 3 5 7 2 5 4 6 2 0 1 0 3 5 7 8 2 5 1 6

   How many 5's in the number? ____________________

   How many 7's in the number? ____________________

   How many 8's in the number? ____________________

   How many 2's in the number? ____________________

   How many 9's in the number? ____________________

---

   b. 3 5 3 8 2 1 9 3 1 9 8 2 6 5 3 9 2 1 5 4 3 8 2 5 4

   How many 0's in the number? ____________________

   How many 3's in the number? ____________________

   How many 7's in the number? ____________________

   How many 8's are followed by 2's? ____________________

   How many 1's are followed by 9's? ____________________

---

   c. 3 6 3 4 7 4 7 7 2 1 3 5 6 7 4 3 9 2 9 5 5 2 3 4 5

   Which number is repeated most often? ____________________

   Which numbers (0–9) are not included? ____________________

   Which numbers are shown four or more times?

   ____

   Which number is listed the least number of times?

   ____

   Circle the numbers surrounded by two numbers that are the same. ____________________

d. 2 5 3 4 5 6 7 6 9 0 3 5 2 4 4 6 7 6 9 9 2 0 1 3 4

How many 7's are surrounded by 6's? ____________________

How many 3's are followed by 4's? ____________________

How many 4's have a number lower than 5 before them?

____

How many numbers are less than 5? ____________________

How many 6's are there? ____________________

---

e. 4 6 3 3 2 3 9 4 3 5 7 7 8 3 8 8 2 8 4 9 0 3 5 4 6

How many 3's and 8's are there altogether?

____

How many numbers are followed by 3's? ____________________

How many 8's are followed by numbers less than 8?

____

How many 8's are there? ____________________

Which number (0–9) is not listed above? ____________________

---

f. 2 1 0 9 8 6 7 2 3 9 0 3 4 5 6 3 2 8 7 6 2 6 3 2

How many 6, 7, and 8's are there altogether?

____

Circle the numbers that are followed by a lower number.

____

How many numbers are below 6? ____________________

If you divide the row of numbers in half, does the left side or the right side have more numbers above 6?

____

Which side has more numbers below 5? ____________________

g. 9 7 8 3 0 2 7 5 5 4 2 0 8 9 6 2 0 8 7 8 9 2 3 5 4

Which number is listed most often? ____________________

Which numbers are listed fewer than three times?

____

Which numbers are listed four times? ____________________

Which number (0–9) is not listed? ____________________

List the numbers that surround the 0's. ____________________

---

h. 5 6 4 4 6 5 9 2 5 6 4 3 6 4

Change each 4 to a 9.

Now how many 4's are there? ____________________

Now how many 9's are there? ____________________

Change each 6 to a 2.

Now how many 2's are there? ____________________

Now how many 3's are there? ____________________

---

i. 2 1 3 4 2 0 3 4 1 2 5 3 2 1

Change each 2 to a 7.

Now how many 7's are there? ____________________

Now how many 2's are there? ____________________

Change each 0 to a 1.

Now how many 1's are there? ____________________

Now how many 3's are there? ____________________

Target Area 4: Numerical Reasoning, Exercise 2

DIRECTIONS: Follow the directions for each question.

1. Answer the following questions on the line provided.

a. 7 3 5 4 3 6 7 3 2 6 3 4 5 9

Change each 6 to a 3, and change each 4 to a 7.

How many 3's are there now? ________

How many 7's are there now? ________

How many 6's are there now? ________

---

b. 3 2 9 0 5 4 8 8 4 5 0 9 2 3

Change each 9 to a 6, change each 5 to a 4, and change each 2 to a 3.

How many 6's are there now? ________

How many 4's are there now? ________

How many 3's are there now? ________

---

c. 7 2 3 1 4 8 2 8 5 2 3 4 7 7

Change each 2 to a 3, and then change each 3 to a 4. Change each 7 to a 6.

How many 3's are there now? ________

How many 4's are there now? ________

How many 6's are there now? ________

---

d. 27 62 45 93 38 46

Which is the next to largest number? ________

Which is the next to smallest number? ________

Which two numbers are closest to each other in value?

____

e. 17 80 47 9 28 52

Which is the next to smallest number? __________

Which is the next to largest number? __________

Which two numbers are farthest apart in value? __________

---

2. Answer the following questions on the lines provided.

a. 71 13 63 33 56 67

Which is the next to largest number? __________

Which is the next to smallest number? __________

Which two numbers are closest to each other in value?

____

---

b. 43 34 52 17 28 76

Which is the next to largest number? __________

Which is the smallest number? __________

Which number is closest to 65? __________

---

c. 35 21 63 52 93 50

Which is the next to largest number? __________

Which two numbers are farthest apart? __________

Which number is closest to 79? __________

---

d. 42 73 10 62 58 83

Which number is farthest from 58? __________

Which two numbers are the smallest? __________

Which number is the second largest? __________

---

e. 210 147 300 163 252 312

Which number is the next to largest? __________

Which number is the next to smallest? __________

Which two numbers are closest to each other? __________

3. Write the correct number on the line provided.

   a. What number is a dozen more than the number of legs a dog has? ________

   b. What number equals the number in a trio plus the number of sides a square has? ________

   c. What number is a decade less than the number of years in a century? ________

   d. What number equals the number of years in a golden wedding anniversary plus the number of pints in a quart? ________

   e. What number equals the number in a duo, the number in an octet, plus the number in a quintet? ________

   f. What number is the same as half the legal voting age?

   ____

   g. What number equals the number of weeks in a year less the number of months in a year? ________

---

4. Fill in the missing numbers in the series.

   Example: 1 2 3 4 _5_ 6 7 _8_

   a. 2 4 6 8 ___ 12 14 ___

   b. 47 46 45 44 ___ 42 41 ___

   c. 11 22 33 44 ___ 66 77 ___

   d. 2 2 4 4 ___ 6 8 ___

   e. 3 13 4 14 ___ 15 6 ___

   f. 10 21 32 43 ___ 65 76 ___

   g. 5 1 5 2 ___ 3 5 ___

   h. 10 1 20 2 ___ 3 40 ___

   i. 3 4 3 5 ___ 6 3 ___

Target Area 4: Listing Steps

DIRECTIONS: Below are different types of activities. There are at least four steps involved in doing each one. On another sheet of paper, write down what you do at each step and list the steps in their proper order. If there are more than four steps, list only the main ones. Each step should be written out as a complete sentence.

EXAMPLE: List four steps in washing a dog.

1. Fill a tub with water.
2. Put the dog in the tub.
3. Wash the dog with soap and water.
4. Rinse the dog thoroughly.

1. List four steps in making a hamburger.
2. List four steps in painting a wall.
3. List four steps in writing a check.
4. List four steps in buying shoes.
5. List four steps to setting a table.
6. List four steps in eating a grapefruit.
7. List four steps to mailing a package.
8. List four steps in cutting hair.
9. List four steps in planning a party.
10. List four steps to mailing a letter.
11. List four steps in making a salad.
12. List four steps in using a coupon.
13. List four steps in buying a birthday present.
14. List four steps in feeding a baby.
15. List four steps in mopping a floor.

16. List four steps in making a bed.
17. List four steps in planning a vacation.
18. List four steps in scrambling an egg.
19. List four steps in defrosting a refrigerator.
20. List four steps in checking out a library book.
21. List four steps in charging a purchase.
22. List four steps in making an ice cream sundae.
23. List four steps in hanging a picture on the wall.
24. List four steps in planting a garden.
25. List four steps in buying a car.
26. List four steps in arranging a picnic.
27. List four steps in going grocery shopping.
28. List four steps in making coffee.
29. List four steps in going to a party.
30. List four steps in fixing a frozen dinner.
31. List four steps in buying an antique.
32. List four steps in polishing a pair of shoes.
33. List four steps in going fishing.
34. List four steps in getting a carry-out meal.
35. List four steps in washing a pan.
36. List four steps in sewing on a button.
37. List four steps in exercising—choose a particular exercise.
38. List four steps in making popcorn.
39. List four steps in getting a plane ticket.
40. List four steps in buying a pet—choose a particular kind of pet.

Target Area 5

USE OF FACTUAL INFORMATION

The aphasic patient often has difficulty recalling information or expressing knowledge he has acquired. In Target Area Five the patient is asked to exercise several different language skills in the performance of tasks requiring the expression of basic information. The exercises are designed for the average adult intelligence; the factual information solicited should be pre-morbid knowledge.

In most of these exercises the patient is asked to answer a question; proper recollection of words and use of syntax will enable him to express his answer. There is latitude for the expression of the patient's own style and personal opinion in this target area. Because patients will vary in the completeness and complexity of their answers to these questions, the clinician may wish to modify the instructions to obtain a particular type of response from an individual patient. This entire series of exercises can be adapted for oral use in group or individual sessions. Target Area Five reflects an important stage in the patient's rehabilitation, the consolidation of all of the language skills he has so far recovered.

M.R.

Target Area 5: Why Questions

DIRECTIONS: On a separate sheet of paper, answer the following questions in complete sentences.

EXAMPLE: Why do people send letters by mail?

It is a quick and inexpensive way to get in touch with someone who is not close by.

1. Why do people use napkins?
2. Why are tape recorders used?
3. Why do some people use alarm clocks?
4. Why do Americans celebrate Veteran's Day?
5. Why are there zoos?
6. Why are there stoplights?
7. Why do most people eat vegetables?
8. Why are banks useful?
9. Why do people get married?
10. Why is there more than one brand of a product at the grocery store?
11. Why is there a federal income tax?
12. Why do we celebrate Labor Day?
13. Why do you need your heart in order to live?
14. Why is gold so expensive?
15. Why is the air polluted?
16. Why are elevators used?
17. Why is it a good idea to be vaccinated?
18. Why is there an American flag?
19. Why is there religion?

20. Why are windows made of glass?
21. Why do we sleep?
22. Why doesn't it snow in southern states?
23. Why do countries have governments?
24. Why do people have pets?
25. Why do fashions change?
26. Why is there a social security program?
27. Why do some people decide to go to college?
28. Why are you answering these questions?
29. Why is it recommended that people wear seat belts?
30. Why do we give aid to foreign countries?
31. Why do people buy insurance?
32. Why do some people take vitamins?
33. Why do many people take photographs?
34. Why do we have many immigrants in this country?
35. Why do trees lose their leaves in the fall?
36. Why do people vote?
37. Why do many women use cosmetics on their faces?
38. Why are there juries at trials?
39. Why do we use calendars?
40. Why are some people opposed to smoking in public places?
41. Why is there a white line painted in the middle of some roads?
42. Why is the United States exploring outer space?
43. Why do people buy lottery tickets?
44. Why do charities need money?
45. Why do we put screens on windows?

Target Area 5: What Questions

DIRECTIONS: On another sheet of paper, answer the following questions fully, completely, and honestly.

EXAMPLE: What is the Fourth of July?

The Fourth of July is a holiday celebrating the birthday of the U.S.

1. What are some duties of policemen?
2. What are the advantages of physical exercise?
3. What is the purpose of newspapers?
4. What is radar?
5. What meal did you eat last and what did you have?
6. What does a real estate agent do?
7. What is the Statue of Liberty?
8. What is the purpose of superhighways?
9. What attractions does your state offer to a tourist?
10. What are maps for?
11. What is an astronaut?
12. What is the purpose of a library?
13. What is extrasensory perception?
14. What are museums for?
15. What is art?
16. What is the purpose of the white lines on a highway?
17. What does a judge do?
18. What is politics?
19. What is the function of a tugboat?
20. What is magic?

21. What is your favorite pastime?
22. What does the word **love** mean to you?
23. What makes you laugh?
24. What do you like least about yourself?
25. What person do you most admire?
26. What is your best quality?
27. What did you do on your last vacation?
28. What makes you mad?
29. What are the names of your family members and their relationship to you?
30. What was the worst thing you ever saw?
31. What was the best thing you ever saw?
32. What was the most unexpected thing that ever happened to you?
33. What was the ugliest thing you ever saw?
34. What was the most beautiful thing you ever saw?
35. What was the most rewarding thing you ever did?
36. What was the happiest thing that ever happened to you?
37. What was the saddest thing that ever happened to you?
38. What was the most embarassing thing that ever happened to you?
39. What was the funniest thing that ever happened to you?
40. What do you feel like right now?
41. What do you want people to remember about you?
42. What do you like doing least each day?
43. What part of the day do you like least?
44. What are you most impatient about?
45. What do you do to relax?

Target Area 5: When Questions

DIRECTIONS: On another sheet of paper, answer the following questions with complete sentences.

EXAMPLE: When is Halloween? Halloween is on October 31.

1. When are newspapers printed?
2. When you're hungry, what do you do?
3. When is the sun in the east?
4. When do leaves change color?
5. When does water freeze?
6. When are you likely to see a rainbow?
7. When would you use a handkerchief?
8. When do you need a road map?
9. When do floods occur?
10. When would you use a flashlight?
11. When do birds fly south?
12. When do we celebrate Independence Day?
13. When does it hail?
14. When do people use sign language?
15. When would someone take an aspirin?
16. When do you use an umbrella?
17. When would someone use a check?
18. When you're bored, what do you do?
19. When are bridges needed?
20. When would you buy stock?
21. When would you be likely to use an antenna?
22. When was World War II?

23. When did Columbus discover America?
24. When are income taxes due?
25. When do you brush your teeth?
26. When you have indigestion, what do you do?
27. When would you defrost a freezer?
28. When would you need a passport?
29. When is it necessary to measure something?
30. When was the last time it rained?
31. When do you think of someone as old?
32. When were "flappers" popular?
33. When is it better to take a bus than to drive a car?
34. When did you wake up this morning?
35. When should you stop at an intersection?
36. When would you use carbon paper?
37. When is it better to use a pencil than a pen?
38. When is your birthday?
39. When would you use a zip code?
40. When do you smile?
41. When are the Olympic Games held?
42. When do you lose your temper?
43. When do you send flowers to someone?
44. When would someone have a hangover?
45. When do license plates expire?

Target Area 5: Where Questions

DIRECTIONS: Answer the following questions in complete sentences on another sheet of paper.

EXAMPLE: Where do you live? *I live on Maple Road in Birmingham, Michigan.*

1. Where would you go to buy a hammer?
2. Where is France?
3. Where is garbage taken?
4. Where do mushrooms grow?
5. Where would you go to buy a kumquat?
6. Where do you put your dirty clothes?
7. Where can you buy newspapers?
8. Where is Florida located?
9. Where is the lake closest to your home?
10. Where can a piano be bought?
11. Where did you go on your last vacation?
12. Where does the sun set in the evening?
13. Where do you live?
14. Where would you go if you were lost?
15. Where do you think your tax money goes?
16. Where does tobacco grow?
17. Where is the Mediterranean Sea?
18. Where could you buy a spark plug?
19. Where is the equator?
20. Where do you register to vote?
21. Where is Niagara Falls located?
22. Where would you find a putting green?

23. Where would you go to find a polar bear?
24. Where does air pollution come from?
25. Where do you do your laundry?
26. Where is San Francisco located?
27. Where could you find sand?
28. Where is Hollywood?
29. Where is Russia?
30. Where are laws made in this country?
31. Where could someone go to get a suntan?
32. Where might someone go to gamble?
33. Where is the best place to buy doughnuts?
34. Where are you now?
35. Where would you go to buy a corsage?
36. Where do you want to go on your next vacation?
37. Where can you find shutters?
38. Where have astronauts traveled?
39. Where would you go to see a volcano?
40. Where could you find a desert?
41. Where are the Rocky Mountains?
42. Where would you buy insect repellent?
43. Where would you go to see a collection of paintings?
44. Where could you keep valuable papers?
45. Where is Rome?

Target Area 5: Who Questions

DIRECTIONS: On another sheet of paper, answer the following questions with complete sentences.

EXAMPLE: Who is Bob Hope? Bob Hope is a comedian.

1. Who is the President of the United States?
2. Who is the Vice President of the United States?
3. Who is the governor of your state?
4. Who was the first President of the United States?
5. Who wrote the Gettysburg Address?
6. Who invented the telephone?
7. Who would you call if you were sick?
8. Who would you go to if your teeth needed cleaning?
9. Who would you see for an eye examination?
10. Who is buried in Grant's tomb?
11. Who can fill prescriptions?
12. Who presides over a trial?
13. Who defends a person who is on trial?
14. Who were the Wright brothers?
15. Who was Winston Churchill?
16. Who was Martin Luther King?
17. Who was Babe Ruth?
18. Who was Albert Einstein?
19. Who is Henry Kissinger?
20. Who were the Beatles?
21. Who discovered electricity?
22. Who was the author of Webster's Dictionary?

23. Who is Mohammed Ali?
24. Who is Elizabeth Taylor?
25. Who developed the Model T?
26. Who is Queen Elizabeth?
27. Who wrote Tom Sawyer and Huckleberry Finn?
28. Who is the First Family?
29. Who is Jerry Falwell?
30. Who was Count Basie?
31. Name a famous woman.
32. Name a famous poet.
33. Name a famous sports personality.
34. Name a famous news commentator.
35. Name an inventor who became famous.
36. Name a famous comedian.
37. Name a famous singer.
38. Name a famous playwright.
39. Name a famous horse.
40. Name a famous explorer.
41. Name a famous fictional character.
42. Name a famous king.
43. Name a famous TV character.
44. Name a famous chef.
45. Name a famous Hollywood star.

Target Area 5: How Questions

DIRECTIONS: Answer the following questions in complete sentences, using another sheet of paper.

EXAMPLE: How do you boil water? *Put water in a pan and put the pan on a burner. Turn the burner to high and wait for the surface of the water to bubble rapidly.*

1. How can you tell whether a peach is ripe?
2. How do you scramble eggs?
3. How can you grow healthy flowers?
4. How could you find out the difference between a real diamond and a fake one?
5. How could you get the names and addresses of all the drugstores in a city?
6. How can you find out which movies are playing in your area?
7. How could you find out what the weather will be like next week?
8. How is a car started?
9. How many inches are in a yard?
10. How much does a gallon of gas cost now?
11. How accurate are opinion polls?
12. How is television different than it was twenty years ago?
13. How often should people eat meals?
14. How many pints are in a quart?
15. How does a microscope make things look larger?
16. How many ounces are in a pound?
17. How could you tell if a piece of bread was stale?

18. How are plate glass and a mirror different?
19. How do secretaries help offices function?
20. How are can openers used?
21. How can you tell if you have a cavity in a tooth?
22. How do you know when to water grass?
23. How do you light a candle?
24. How do you change your order in a restaurant?
25. How do you polish shoes?
26. How do you change a lightbulb?
27. How can you tell whether a house needs a new coat of paint?
28. How can you show someone you like him or her?
29. How do you make a sandwich?
30. How can you tell when it's safe to cross the street?
31. How is a long distance phone call made?
32. How can you tell if it is going to rain?
33. How do you show anger?
34. How can you tell the difference between a weed and a plant?
35. How are francs, pesos, and guineas alike?
36. How would you explain what marijuana is?
37. How can you locate a doctor?
38. How do you know if someone is telling the truth?
39. How can you tell if someone has a sunburn?
40. How do you brush your teeth?
41. How can you tell if a hamburger is cooked enough to eat?
42. How can you tell if an animal has fleas?
43. How do you eat an orange?
44. How do you know if you need to have your hair cut?
45. How do you know if a watch is keeping the correct time?

Target Area 5: General Facts, Exercise 1

DIRECTIONS: Fill in the blanks with the correct answer.

EXAMPLE: A square has *four* ______________ sides.

1. A triangle has ______________ sides.
2. A carpenter works with ______________.
3. Venus is a ______________.
4. A year has ______________ months.
5. The north-south dividing line of the earth is the ______________.
6. A pancreas can be found in ______________.
7. Independence Day is ______________.
8. A tuba is a(n) ______________.
9. A holiday after Labor Day is ______________.
10. An Academy Award is given for ______________.
11. The animal that carries her young in a pouch is called a ______________.
12. A person who leases land or houses is a ______________.
13. 17% is written out as ______________.
14. Two types of fasteners for clothes are ______________ and ______________.
15. An organ is ______________.
16. The caboose is the ______________ car on a train.

    baggage   first   dining   last

17. Mechanics ______________ cars.
18. The U.S. Congress consists of the ______________ and the ______________.

19. ______________________ is a state west of the Mississippi River.

20. When snow melts it becomes ______________________ .

21. The place where two streets cross is called an

______________________ .

22. Agriculture has to do with ______________________ .

23. The Amish are ______________________ .

24. A ______________________ is a place where prescriptions are filled.

25. A colon looks like ______________________ .

? “ : ;

26. A zip code refers to ______________________ .

27. Pacemakers are used for ______________________ .

28. An interstate highway goes ______________________ .

north and south between states in one state

four lanes through all national parks

29. Bought rhymes with ______________________ .

tough caught bout dot

30. Another word for shrub is ______________________ .

31. A jockey is a ______________________ .

32. Bach and Beethoven were both ______________________ .

33. Someone from Paris is called a ______________________ .

34. Chili con carne is ______________________ .

35. Ocean tides are caused by the moon. True or False?

____

36. The other half of Tweedledum is

______________________ .

37. The female counterpart of a rooster is a ______________________.

38. A shelter for pigs is called a ______________________.

39. A puck is used in what sport? ______________________

40. Beagles are ______________________.

41. If you were in a greenhouse, what would you be looking at?

____

42. Name a well-known board game. ______________________

43. A comic strip is drawn by a ______________________.

44. When does one receive a pension? ______________________

45. You would see an obituary in a ______________________.

46. Check all the things you would use for an outdoor barbecue.

_____ concrete _____ fertilizer _____ grill

_____ charcoal _____ utensils _____ plates

47. How are earn and urn alike? ______________________

48. ______________________ is used between bricks to seal them together.

49. ______________________ is the capital of ______________________.

50. An illustrated book means that it has ______________________.

Target Area 5: General Facts, Exercise 2

DIRECTIONS: Answer the following questions with complete sentences. Use another sheet of paper.

EXAMPLE: What is a potholder? A pot holder is a piece of heavy material. People use potholders to protect their hands when handling something hot.

1. Who was Harry Truman?
2. When do you use an area code?
3. What is a cube?
4. What is lumber?
5. Why is an object polished?
6. A desert is different from a dessert. How?
7. Who was the first person to land on the moon?
8. What is high blood pressure?
9. Where are bananas grown?
10. How do you get a driver's license?
11. What is a cannibal?
12. Where is the Riviera?
13. Where is gambling legal in the United States?
14. How old do you have to be before you can vote?
15. What is stereophonic sound?
16. Is a souffle something to build?
17. What is a stroke?
18. What is an old wives' tale?
19. Why might you need an accountant?
20. What makes up an orchestra?

21. Name an animal that can see better in the night than in the day.
22. What does a stenographer do?
23. What is chain smoking?
24. What makes a person an alcoholic?
25. Where would you find a popsicle?
26. What is a sense of humor?
27. How long is an eternity?
28. What are the names of these shapes? 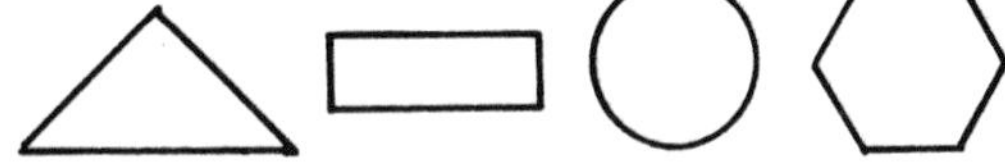
29. What is a tow truck used for?
30. What is a prophet?
31. Where were you born?
32. What is the Rose Bowl game?
33. What is Sears Roebuck?
34. Why was Billy the Kid famous?
35. What kind of training does a doctor need to have?
36. When is a woman referred to as a widow?
37. What is a cockatoo?
38. Why do people sometimes have rummage sales?
39. What is a Toyota?
40. How do you finance a purchase?
41. What is a median?
42. Why do dogs pant?
43. Name a serious disease.
44. Where do you keep cheese?
45. What can make you sneeze?

Target Area 6

USE OF CONCRETE REASONING

When language loss occurs, the necessary reasoning processes can be affected and the patient's ability to reason by an orderly progression to a rational conclusion is sometimes lost or impaired. The aphasic patient may sometimes use factual information inappropriately or stray from relevancy. Thus an individual's response inadvertently moves away from its logical end.

Target Area Six is concerned with strengthening deductive, concrete reasoning abilities. Some of the exercises offer a choice of answers, while others specify that a complete phrase or sentence must be written. All of the exercises may be modified for work on receptive language skills for the patient having auditory comprehension difficulty or a reduced auditory retention span. Many of the following exercises can easily be modified to provide even more complex reasoning tasks.

M.R.

Target Area 6: Yes or No

DIRECTIONS: Answer **yes** or **no** to the following questions. Write the answer in the blank below the question.

EXAMPLE: Can you sip milk? yes

1. Can you eat a lemon?
   ____
2. Can you saddle a flea?
   ____
3. Can you polish a car?
   ____
4. Can you order a telephone?
   ____
5. Can you collect a spider?
   ____
6. Can you bite a canoe?
   ____
7. Can you erase chalk?
   ____
8. Can you postpone a lid?
   ____
9. Can you hop on your head?
   ____
10. Can you walk on ice?
    ____
11. Can you bake a typewriter?
    ____
12. Can you mop with mosquitoes?
    ____
13. Can you buy thumbs?
    ____
14. Can you send flowers?
    ____
15. Can you eat a banjo?
    ____
16. Can you celebrate paper?
    ____
17. Can you climb a trellis?
    ____
18. Can you crawl on sand?
    ____
19. Can vegetables be chopped?
    ____
20. Can foam float?
    ____
21. Can you paint eagles?
    ____
22. Can you entertain an omelette?
    ____

23. Can you travel in a surrey?

____

24. Can you hit hydrogen?

____

25. Can scales be sung?

____

26. Can you buy calculus?

____

27. Can syllables be articulated?

____

28. Can binoculars be adjusted?

____

29. Can you excavate minerals?

____

30. Can novels pucker?

____

31. Can camels imbibe?

____

32. Can computers calculate?

____

33. Can artifacts break?

____

34. Can decanters smell?

____

35. Can torches illuminate?

____

36. Can licenses be revoked?

____

37. Can pizzas perspire?

____

38. Can odometers smell?

____

39. Can attorneys judge?

____

40. Can beauticians cut hair?

____

41. Can measles be infectious?

____

42. Can submarines verify?

____

43. Can woodpeckers sting?

____

44. Can physicians operate?

____

45. Can subscriptions expire?

____

46. Can canines chew?

____

47. Can canteens be eaten?

____

48. Can caterpillars fly?

____

49. Can patios be stolen?

____

50. Can cats be neutered?

____

Target Area 6: Which One

DIRECTIONS: Read the question and circle the correct answer.

EXAMPLE: Which is a day of the week? January or Thursday

1. Which would you use to hang a picture on a wall?

   a staple or a nail

2. Which would you use to cut paper?

   a scissors or a knife

3. Which would you use to hem a dress?

   string or thread

4. Which would you use to light a fire?

   a match or charcoal

5. Which would you use to protect your hands?

   detergent or gloves

6. Which would you use for a headache?

   a decongestant or an aspirin

7. Which would you use when you're hot?

   a blanket or a fan

8. Which would you use if you couldn't see well?

   glasses or a hearing aid

9. Which would you use to clean a window?

   Exlax or Windex

10. Which would you use to measure distances?

    an inch or a pint

11. Which would you use if you were weeding?

    a hoe or a shovel

12. Which would you use to catch a baseball?

    a mitt or a mitten

13. Which is bigger? a bicycle or a boat
14. Which is smaller? a lemon or a typewriter
15. Which is bigger? a pen or a pin
16. Which is bigger? a bell or a piano
17. Which is smaller? a football or a baseball
18. Which is bigger? a pizza or a pickle
19. Which is smaller? a slide projector or a motel
20. Which is smaller? a plate or a saucer
21. Which is bigger? a postmark or a postcard
22. Which is smaller? a Saint Bernard or a poodle
23. Which is bigger? a bush or a tree
24. Which is bigger? a magazine or a newspaper
25. Which is smaller? a chair or a stool
26. Which is bigger? a calf or a kitten
27. Which is smaller? an olive or an apple
28. Which is smaller? a bracelet or an earring
29. Which is bigger? a golf ball or a tennis ball
30. Which is bigger? a tongue or a tooth
31. Which is smaller? an onion or a radish
32. Which is smaller? a yardstick or a ruler
33. Which is bigger? a violin or a guitar
34. Which is smaller? a pear or a raisin
35. Which is bigger? a hamster or a panda
36. Which is bigger? a worm or a snake
37. Which is smaller? a pond or an ocean
38. Which is bigger? a pigeon or a pig

39. Which is heavier? an organ or a glass of milk
40. Which is lighter? a hamburger or a meatloaf
41. Which is lighter? a cigarette or an ashtray
42. Which is heavier? a train or a sofa
43. Which is lighter? a chandelier or a guinea pig
44. Which is heavier? a pound of lead or a pound of feathers
45. Which is heavier? a gallon of gas or a quart of gas
46. Which is lighter? an elephant or a bookcase
47. Which is lighter? whipped cream or mashed potatoes
48. Which is heavier? a telephone or a bed
49. Which is heavier? a blanket or a sheet
50. Which is heavier? thread or rope
51. Which is lighter? a bottle of wine or a can of beer
52. Which is heavier? a rock or a shell
53. Which is lighter? a paper plate or a china plate
54. Which is lighter? a balloon or a basketball
55. Which is heavier? a bowl or a statue
56. Which is lighter? a card table or a deck of cards
57. Which is heavier? a horseshoe or a horsefly
58. Which is heavier? an overcoat or a sweater
59. Which is lighter? a camera or a photograph
60. Which is heavier? an alarm clock or a watch
61. Which is lighter? a sock or a shoe
62. Which is lighter? a bicycle or a motorcycle
63. Which is heavier? you or your shadow
64. Which is lighter? sunglasses or field glasses

65. Which comes first? dinner or breakfast
66. Which comes last? 317 or 371
67. Which comes last? the follower or the leader
68. Which comes first? lightning or thunder
69. Which comes last? the voice or the echo
70. Which comes last? the conclusion or the introduction
71. Which comes last? Halloween or Easter
72. Which comes first? the wound or the scar
73. Who came last? Adam or Eve
74. Which comes first? the chicken or the egg
75. Which comes first? the wine or the grape
76. Which comes last? the dough or the cookie
77. Which comes last? grade school or high school
78. Which comes last? a fawn or a doe
79. Which comes first? a bud or a flower
80. Which comes first? ice or water
81. Which comes last? a blueprint or a house
82. Which comes first? a shampoo or a set
83. Which comes first? salad or dessert
84. Which comes last? aspirin or a headache
85. Which comes last? Thanksgiving or Christmas
86. Which comes first? opening night or rehearsal
87. Which comes last? birth or death
88. Which comes last? pregnancy or a baby
89. Which comes first? an invitation or a party
90. Which comes last? a caterpillar or a butterfly

Target Area 6: Reasonable Conclusions

DIRECTIONS: Complete the sentences below in a logical way.

EXAMPLE: Plants need water because *it is their food and they would die without it.*

1. Some people prefer to travel by plane rather than by car because

____

____

2. Safety belts are worn in cars because

____

____

3. It's a good idea to rest when you're sick because

____

____

4. Sunglasses are worn because

____

____

5. People like to eat in restaurants because

____

____

6. Many people turn off the lights when they leave a room because

____

____

7. Large cities are usually found near a body of water because

____

____

8. People use canes because

____

____

9. Most people wear socks or stockings because

____

____

10. Dieting is popular because

____

____

11. Many people go on vacations because

____

____

12. Bandages are used on cuts because

____

____

13. Companies give out free samples of products because

____

____

14. Research and experiments are carried on because

____

____

15. Hospitals sterilize instruments because

____

____

16. Banks have drive-in windows because

____

____

17. Cats lick themselves because

____

____

18. Fresh food is better than processed food because

____

____

19. A telephone book provides Yellow Pages because

____

____

20. Many people use credit cards because

____

____

21. Coal is cheaper than oil because

____

____

22. Women carry purses because

____

____

23. Stores have sales because

____

____

24. Television shows have commercials because

____

____

25. People take baths because

____

____

26. Policemen wear guns because

____

____

27. Many businessmen make reservations before they travel because

____

____

28. Religion is important to some people because

____

____

29. Professional athletes receive high salaries because

____

____

30. Lawbreakers are punished because

____

____

31. Most people have locks on their doors because

____

____

32. It is important for citizens to vote because

____

____

33. Some people are vegetarians because

____

____

34. People get magazine subscriptions because

____

____

35. Stairs have railings because

____

____

36. People wear hearing aids because

____

____

37. Streets have traffic lights because

____

____

38. Some people play the lottery because

____

____

Target Area 6: Similarities and Differences, Exercise 1

DIRECTIONS: Answer the following questions by explaining what the two items have **in common.** Use a separate sheet of paper.

EXAMPLE: What are two ways that a dog and a cat are alike?

a. They are both pets.

b. They both have four legs.

1. What are two ways that a pen and a pencil are alike?
2. What are two ways a motorcycle and a bicycle are alike?
3. What are two ways March and May are alike?
4. What are two ways a governor and a mayor are alike?
5. What are two ways a boat and a ship are alike?
6. What are two ways a flower and a tree are alike?
7. What are two ways a mouse and a rat are alike?
8. What are two ways a boy and a man are alike?
9. What are two ways toenails and fingernails are alike?
10. What are two ways a piano and an organ are alike?
11. What are two ways brownies and cookies are alike?
12. What are two ways France and Switzerland are alike?
13. What are two ways college and high school are alike?
14. What are two ways diamonds and rubies are alike?
15. What are two ways a quarter and a dime are alike?
16. What are two ways a tiger and a lion are alike?
17. What are two ways an orange and a tangerine are alike?
18. What are two ways a cocker spaniel and a poodle are alike?
19. What are two ways spring and fall are alike?
20. What are two ways radio and television are alike?

Target Area 6: Similarities and Differences, Exercise 2

DIRECTIONS: Answer the following questions by explaining how the items are **different.** Use a separate sheet of paper.

EXAMPLE: What are two ways a dog and a cat are different?

a. A dog barks, but a cat meows.

b. A cat can climb a tree, but a dog can't.

1. What are two ways an apple and a banana are different?
2. What are two ways a kite and an airplane are different?
3. What are two ways a dollar bill and a quarter are different?
4. What are two ways a clock and a watch are different?
5. What are two ways gloves and mittens are different?
6. What are two ways a sweater and a coat are different?
7. What are two ways corn and lettuce are different?
8. What are two ways crayons and chalk are different?
9. What are two ways an apple tree and pine tree are different?
10. What are two ways a Pontiac and a Volkswagen are different?
11. What are two ways a lawyer and a jury are different?
12. What are two ways whipped cream and sour cream are different?
13. What are two ways an orange and a grapefruit are different?
14. What are two ways a chipmunk and a squirrel are different?
15. What are two ways rings and necklaces are different?
16. What are two ways the sun and the moon are different?
17. What are two ways a novel and a dictionary are different?
18. What are two ways Wednesday and Sunday are different?
19. What are two ways a football and a baseball are different?
20. What are the two ways that squares and triangles are different?

Target Area 6: Main Differences

DIRECTIONS: Complete each sentence below by explaining the **main** difference between the two items. There probably are several differences, but only write about the one that seems to be the **most important** difference.

EXAMPLE: The main difference between a **bear** and a **robin** is that a robin can fly, but a bear can't.

1. The main difference between a **telephone** and a **telegram** is ______________________________

2. The main difference between a **pen** and a **pencil** is ______________________________

3. The main difference between **cream** and **skim milk** is ______________________________

4. The main difference between a **spoon** and a **knife** is ______________________________

5. The main difference between a **cup** and a **glass** is ______________________________

6. The main difference between a **tricycle** and a **bicycle** is

____

____

7. The main difference between a **circle** and a **square** is

____

____

8. The main difference between **fore** and **four** is

____

____

9. The main difference between **tennis** and **badminton** is

____

____

10. The main difference between a **vest** and a **sweater** is

____

____

11. The main difference between **shoes** and **boots** is

____

____

12. The main difference between a **nurse** and a **doctor** is

____

____

13. The main difference between a **book** and a **magazine** is

____

____

14. The main difference between **tea** and **coffee** is

____

____

15. The main difference between a **purse** and a **suitcase** is

____

____

16. The main difference between a **lamp** and a **flashlight** is

____

____

17. The main difference between **ice cream** and **sherbet** is

____

____

18. The main difference between a **sedan** and a **station wagon** is

____

____

19. The main difference between a **drugstore** and a **hardware store** is

____

____

20. The main difference between a **cherry** and a **watermelon** is

____

____

21. The main difference between **clay** and **mud** is

____

____

22. The main difference between a **button** and a **zipper** is

____

____

23. The main difference between a **necklace** and a **scarf** is

____

____

24. The main difference between a **screw** and a **nail** is

____

____

25. The main difference between **yesterday** and **tomorrow** is

____

____

26. The main difference between **television** and **radio** is

____

____

27. The main difference between **checkers** and **chess** is

____

____

28. The main difference between a **screen** and a **window** is

____

____

29. The main difference between a **trailer** and a **motor home** is

____

____

30. The main difference between a **megaphone** and a **microphone** is

____

____

31. The main difference between a **chair** and a **couch** is

____

____

32. The main difference between a **paper bag** and a **plastic bag** is

____

____

33. The main difference between a **horse** and a **colt** is

____

____

34. The main difference between a **mirror** and **glass** is

____

____

35. The main difference between **toast** and **bread** is

____

____

36. The main difference between **gray** and **black** is

____

____

37. The main difference between a **cane** and **crutches** is

____

____

38. The main difference between a **snack** and a **meal** is

____

____

39. The main difference between a **barber** and a **beautician** is

____

____

40. The main difference between an **ocean** and a **lake** is

____

____

41. The main difference between **grass** and **weeds** is

____

____

42. The main difference between **sugar** and **nutra-sweet** is

____

____

43. The main difference between a **trunk** and a **suitcase** is

____

____

44. The main difference between a **plant** and **cut flowers** is

____

____

45. The main difference between a **chair** and a **stool** is

____

____

Target Area 6: Constant Characteristics, Exercise 1

DIRECTIONS: Read the sentence and circle the correct answer. The answer is the one that is **always** associated with each item, not just some of the time. There is only one correct answer for each question.

EXAMPLE: A pen **always** has

blue ink   ink   a clip   an eraser

1. A lake **always** has

   weeds   water   fish   a dam

2. A telephone **always** has

   a busy signal   buttons   a dial   a receiver

3. A book **always** has

   chapters   pages   pictures   index

4. A sailboat **always** has

   a galley   sails   a motor   oars

5. A pencil **always** has

   a sharp point   an eraser   a wooden outside   lead

6. A desk **always** has

   a flat surface   cubbyholes   a blotter   drawers

7. A fish **always** has

   gills   teeth   4 fins   eyelids

8. A farm **always** has

   cows   a barn   soil   flowers

9. A baseball team **always** has

a ball gloves a mascot nine members

---

10. A newspaper **always** has

an editor a woman's section

horoscopes an evening edition

---

11. An automobile **always** has

a convertible top bucket seats tires two doors

---

12. A rose bush **always** has

roots flowers a pot green leaves

---

13. A house **always** has

a roof a basement a dining room a porch

---

14. A typewriter **always** has

carbon paper keys red type a secretary

---

15. A man's suit **always** has

a vest cuffs a tie a jacket

---

16. Shoes **always** have

soles laces heels buckles

---

17. A mountain **always** has

streams a snow cap height trees

---

18. A steak **always**

has a bone is meat is a sirloin is from a cow

---

19. A doctor **always**

operates makes a lot of money

cures people is educated

20. A dog **always** has

long hair puppies a collar paws

21. An apple **always** has

a worm red skin a core bruises

22. A chair **always** has

upholstery a back a seat arms

23. A television **always** has

color an antenna channels soap operas

24. A portrait **always** has

colors scenery a subject a frame

25. Eyeglasses **always**

have cases improve vision are bifocals have lenses

26. A guitar **always** has

eight strings a pick catgut strings

27. A rainbow **always**

has a pot of gold has color

lasts fifteen minutes is orange

28. A mirror **always**

reflects has a frame

hangs on a wall needs cleaning

29. A helicopter **always**

has wings carries passengers

lands at airports has propellers

30. On your birthday you **always** get

presents   older   a cake   cards

---

31. A kitchen **always**

is where you eat   has a dishwasher

has linoleum   has a sink

---

32. A clock **always**

has a second hand   tells time

has twelve numbers on it   ticks

---

33. A waterfall **always** has

water   moss   foam   a rainbow

---

34. Cheddar cheese **always** is

yellow   a dairy product   soft   imported

---

35. Stars **always** are

white   planets   far from earth   the same size

---

36. A bicycle **always** has

a rider   a horn   a seat   a basket

---

37. Communication **always**

is verbal   gives a message

is understood   is between people

---

38. A flag **always** is

a symbol   red, white, and blue

on a flagpole   made of cloth

---

39. A library **always** has

tapes   information   records   periodicals

Target Area 6: Constant Characteristics, Exercise 2

DIRECTIONS: Complete the questions below by answering with what is **always** true for each item. The answer should be something that is **always** associated with each item.

EXAMPLE: Dogs always have four legs.

1. An elephant always ______________________________
____

2. A cantalope always ______________________________
____

3. A dictionary always ______________________________
____

4. A ball always ______________________________
____

5. A tape recorder always ______________________________
____

6. Paper always ______________________________
____

7. A year always ______________________________
____

8. A profile always ______________________________
____

9. The President always ______________________________
____

10. California always ______________________________

____

11. Oatmeal cookies always ______________________________

____

12. Screwdrivers always ______________________________

____

13. Restaurants always ______________________________

____

14. Cars always ______________________________

____

15. Lawyers always ______________________________

____

16. Calendars always ______________________________

____

17. Jackets always ______________________________

____

18. Paintbrushes always ______________________________

____

19. Whales always ______________________________

____

20. Tables always ______________________________

____

21. Eggs always ______________________________
____

22. Airplanes always ______________________________
____

23. Violins always ______________________________
____

24. A rose always ______________________________
____

25. Lobsters always ______________________________
____

26. A canoe always ______________________________
____

27. A spoon always ______________________________
____

28. Teeth always ______________________________
____

29. Glue always ______________________________
____

30. Forks always ______________________________
____

Target Area 6: Commonalities, Exercise

DIRECTIONS: In each group of five words below, there is one word which does not belong with the others. Cross out that word. On the line, write another word that fits into the group.

EXAMPLE: cat dog ~~handle~~ horse tiger

bear
____

1. sofa chair coffee table cup desk

____

2. scrambled stamped poached fried hard boiled

____

3. nickel dime peso quarter penny

____

4. Robert Linda Susan Carol Diane

____

5. orange banana pineapple lemon potato

____

6. stream strain strike porch strong

____

7. Chevrolet Jaguar Pontiac Ford Dodge

____

8. funny cloudy sunny overcast stormy

____

9. Time Bible Newsweek People Life

____

10. one way stop open yield do not enter

____

11. celery lettuce soup tomato cucumber

____

12. As the World Turns Sound of Music My Fair Lady Oklahoma Camelot ____________________

13. perch tuna clam salmon bass

____

14. ringmaster clocks acrobats lion tamer clowns

____

15. cap bonnet helmet socks beret

____

16. poinsettia ivy philodendron cactus tomato

____

17. pine oak walnut mahogany peanut

____

18. pants sweater turtleneck vest blouse

____

19. emerald diamond ruby pearls sapphire

____

20. cups wine glasses mugs goblets

____

21. tug airplane raft yacht canoe

____

22. France Germany India Italy Spain

____

23. triangles circles squares rectangles lines

____

24. tabby poodle beagle spaniel collie

____

25. gin water Scotch whiskey rum

____

26. piano violin song trumpet organ

____

27. legs bones arms shoulders feet

____

28. calf puppy lamb kitten goat

____

29. iced tea lemonade coffee milkshake ice cream soda

____

30. veal beef lamb pork shrimp

____

31. leaves twigs lumber sticks wood

____

32. pal friend buddy boss chum

____

33. murder robbery assault attack accident

____

34. diapers cologne bottle pacifier layette

____

35. square box circle rectangle cube

____

36. Jesus Catholic Jewish Buddhist Baptist

____

37. bottle lantern flashlight chandelier candle

____

38. drawer carton suitcase tray crate

____

Target Area 6: Commonalities, Exercise 2

DIRECTIONS: The four words in each group have something in common. Explain what they have in common without using one of the listed words. Write a complete sentence.

EXAMPLE: cat dog bird horse

They are all animals.

1. fourteen seventy-five thirty two

2. eyes nose mouth cheeks

3. Treasure Island Heidi Tom Sawyer Alice in Wonderland

4. winter summer spring autumn

5. stream lake river ocean

6. palette brush canvas easel

7. Colby Cheddar mozzarella Swiss

8. George Henry Robert James

9. weeping willow maple sycamore oak

10. sandals boots slippers sneakers

11. granite quartz calcite marble

12. pie cookies cake doughnuts

13. Fourth of July Labor Day Thanksgiving Christmas

14. street road avenue boulevard

15. baseball hockey football basketball

16. azure turquoise navy aquamarine

17. aspirin cough drops laxatives sedatives

18. spaghetti antipasto spumoni lasagna

19. cinnamon pepper cloves nutmeg

20. governor mayor county clerk judge

21. jet blimp helicopter airplane

22. camera film dark room lens

23. staples paper clips tape glue

24. arithmetic reading spelling writing

25. screen antenna knobs volume dial

26. Saskatchewan Ontario Nova Scotia Quebec

27. Time Ladies Home Journal Sports Illustrated Saturday Evening Post

28. John Adams Grover Cleveland Andrew Jackson Zachary Taylor

29. mosquitoes dragonflies gnats spiders

30. fingernail thumb knuckle palm

31. cardinal wren thrush crow

32. bonds Wall Street market index dividends

33. Bob Hope Jack Benny Milton Berle Don Rickles

34. Bahamas Jamaica Virgin Islands Aruba

35. Appalachians Alps Himalayas Rockies

36. calcium iron magnesium potassium

37. cabin cottage lodge trailer

38. deck patio porch veranda

Target Area 6: Ordering of Events, Exercise 1

DIRECTIONS: The following sentences tell a short story, but they have been put into the wrong order. Number the sentences 1–6 so that what happens first is number 1, what happens last is number 6, and all of the sentences are in the right order.

EXAMPLE:

5 Pick the book up off the shelf.

2 Ask the librarian where the science books are.

6 Open the book.

3 Walk to the science section.

1 Walk into the library.

4 Look for the book that you want.

1. __ Tie a single knot.

   __ Loosen the shoe laces and pull the tongue up.

   __ Pull the loops through and tie the bow.

   __ Put one finger on the knot and make a loop around another finger.

   __ Put the shoe on your foot.

   __ Hold a lace in each hand and pull tightly.

---

2. __ Pour the filling into the pie.

   __ Set the timer on the oven.

   __ Roll out the pie crust and form it in the plate.

   __ Put the pie into the hot oven.

   __ Get out all the ingredients to be used.

   __ Prepare the pie filling.

3. ___ Fasten the seat belt.

___ Turn the ignition key and press the accelerator.

___ Drive down the road.

___ Put the car in gear.

___ Open the car door and get in.

___ Put the key in the ignition.

---

4. ___ Leave for home.

___ Arrive at the party.

___ Respond to the invitation.

___ Spend the evening at the party.

___ Dress for the party.

___ Open the invitation.

---

5. ___ Address envelope.

___ Put the letter in the envelope.

___ Get out a pen and paper.

___ Put a stamp on the envelope.

___ Write a letter to your friend.

___ Put the letter in the mail.

---

6. ___ I ate a hearty breakfast.

___ I woke up early with the sun shining through the windows.

___ I got dressed in my work clothes.

___ It was a beautiful fall morning.

___ Now I could go outdoors.

___ I opened the garage door and got out my rake.

7. ___ Carry on a conversation.

___ Dial the number.

___ Pick up the receiver.

___ Listen for the dial tone.

___ Ask for the person to whom you wish to speak.

___ Say goodbye and hang up the phone.

---

8. ___ The month of weddings and graduations

___ The beginning of spring

___ The month with Christmas

___ The month of Valentine's Day

___ The month of Independence Day

___ The beginning of fall

---

9. ___ Boil the spaghetti for 10 minutes.

___ Put the spaghetti and some sauce on the plate.

___ Drain the spaghetti.

___ Measure out the spaghetti.

___ Put the spaghetti in the water.

___ Boil water in a large pot.

---

10. ___ She straightened the paper.

___ She signed the letter.

___ She typed the letter.

___ She pulled the paper out of the typewriter.

___ She placed the paper on the roll and rotated it.

___ She set the margins on each side.

11. ___ Write the date on the check.

___ Fill in the amount of money.

___ Get out your check book.

___ Sign your name to the check.

___ Mail the check.

___ Write the name of the person you're paying.

---

12. ___ He pushed the button and waited for the elevator.

___ He moved to the rear as more people got on.

___ He got out of the elevator.

___ He said "out, please" when the elevator reached his floor.

___ He pushed the button for the floor he wanted.

___ The elevator arrived and he stepped in.

---

13. ___ I closed the box with the vase in it.

___ I folded the paper around the box and taped it together.

___ I placed the vase in the box.

___ I wrapped the vase in tissue paper.

___ I cut wrapping paper to fit around the box.

___ I made a bow and placed it on top.

---

14. ___ She scooped the ice cream out and put it in a dish.

___ She removed the ice cream from the freezer.

___ Her husband poured sauce over the ice cream.

___ He placed the cherry on top.

___ He squirted on the whipped cream.

___ She put the ice cream back in the freezer.

15. ___ When I opened the door I saw it was a beautiful day.

___ After brushing my teeth, I went downstairs.

___ I stretched and yawned before getting out of bed.

___ I plugged in the coffee and went to get the paper.

___ The alarm rang at exactly seven o'clock.

___ Then I jumped out of bed and put on a robe.

---

16. ___ Hit the ball!

___ Wait for the right pitch.

___ Try a few practice swings.

___ Stand in position ready to hit.

___ Choose your bat.

___ Take your place at home plate.

---

17. ___ Look at a few different models and styles.

___ Find a salesperson to talk with.

___ Ask the salesperson any questions you have.

___ Visit the showroom for that car.

___ Take a test drive.

___ Decide what kind of car you would like to buy.

---

18. ___ I am sitting at my desk.

___ The phone is off the hook and I don't expect any visitors.

___ I put a clean sheet of paper in my trusty typewriter.

___ I've been sitting here for 15 minutes with no ideas.

___ Today I will begin to write the great American novel.

___ At last—an inspiration! "Once upon a time. . . ."

Target Area 6: Ordering of Events, Exercise 2

DIRECTIONS: To answer each of the questions below, put the sentences in the right order. What happens first is number 1 and what happens last is number 6.

1. If you were on a picnic and wanted to grill hamburgers, in what order would you do the following things?

__ Light the fire.

__ Look for wood for the fire.

__ Put the hamburgers on the grill.

__ Place the grill over the fire.

__ Turn the hamburgers over.

__ Stack kindling and newspaper in a cleared area.

---

2. If you were going to plant a garden, in what order would you do the following things?

__ Buy seeds for the garden.

__ Plant the seeds.

__ Dig up the ground.

__ Weed the garden.

__ Decide where to put the garden.

__ Add fertilizer to the ground.

3. If you were going to take a shower, in what order would you do the following?

    ___ Turn on the water.

    ___ Test the water for the right temperature.

    ___ Get in the shower.

    ___ Rinse off the soap.

    ___ Take off your clothes.

    ___ Wash with soap.

---

4. If you wanted to watch television, in what order would you do the following?

    ___ Adjust the volume.

    ___ Find the TV guide.

    ___ Sit down and watch the program.

    ___ Check to see what programs are on.

    ___ Adjust the picture so that it's clear.

    ___ Turn on the TV.

---

5. If you wanted to take a dog for a walk, in what order would you do the following?

    ___ Attach the leash to the dog's collar.

    ___ Call the dog.

    ___ Open the door and go out.

    ___ Grip the leash securely in your hand.

    ___ Stop at trees.

    ___ Get out the leash.

6. If you wanted to paint a picture, in what order would you do the following?

    ___ Decide what you want to paint and make a sketch.

    ___ Put in shadowing and highlights.

    ___ Tack canvas onto the easel.

    ___ Assemble your paints and brushes.

    ___ Lightly put in the background and the basics.

    ___ Add the finishing touches.

---

7. ___ He can usually cover fifty to seventy-five feet in one gliding jump.

    ___ As he glides, he also uses his tail to guide him.

    ___ The flying squirrel is a small, unusual kind of squirrel.

    ___ He has extra folds of skin on each side of his body.

    ___ When he flies, these folds act like gliding wings.

    ___ These folds connect his front and back legs.

---

8. ___ After his marriage he was rehired as leader of the Marine Band.

    ___ A few years later he quit the band and toured the country with variety shows.

    ___ While he was leader of the band he wrote many of his famous marches.

    ___ When John Philip Sousa was thirteen he became an apprentice in the Marine Band.

    ___ At twenty-five he married a girl from Philadelphia.

    ___ Probably his most famous march is "Stars and Stripes Forever."

9. ___ Jesse James was born in 1847.

___ The townspeople fought them and killed all but Jesse and his brother.

___ To escape the governor, Jesse moved and called himself Tom Howard.

___ One year later, in 1882, he was killed by Robert Ford.

___ In 1876 he and seven other men tried to rob a bank in Minnesota.

___ In 1881 the Governor of Missouri offered a reward for either Frank or Jesse.

---

10. ___ He then transferred to the University of Southern California, where he won the Heisman Trophy for being the best college player in the nation.

___ While he was there, he was named junior college All-American twice.

___ O. J. Simpson is a nationally known football player.

___ After that he joined the Buffalo Bills, a professional football team.

___ But it's usually not known that as a child he was the leader of a street gang.

___ Because his high school grades weren't very good he attended a junior college.

11. ___ It is located in a large mall in Washington D.C.
 ___ In addition to the Smithsonian, the mall includes six other cultural buildings.
 ___ The Smithsonian is also a research center and has as many teachers as a large university.
 ___ The newest building in the complex is the National Air and Space Museum.
 ___ In 1976 over twenty million people visited the more than thirty-five acres of displays in its eleven halls.
 ___ The Smithsonian Institution is the largest museum in the world.

---

12. ___ This means some people can safely drink three one-ounce drinks of one hundred proof whiskey a day.
 ___ The effect of too much alcohol in the system can be harmful.
 ___ Researchers have defined a "safe" level of drinking.
 ___ Drinking more than this amount is not considered safe.
 ___ This equals one and a half ounces of pure alcohol.
 ___ This is also equivalent to four eight-ounce glasses of beer or half of a bottle of wine.

---

13. ___ The final step is doing a travel stroke to move you toward help or shore.
 ___ Drownproofing is a way of saving these lives.
 ___ The first step is finding a position that lets you float, then you do a stroke that helps you breathe.
 ___ Experts say that 95% of these deaths could have been avoided.
 ___ Each year roughly eight thousand Americans drown.
 ___ There are three basic steps to drownproofing.

14. ___ Their first defense was their location.

___ Their second defense was the moat around them.

___ Finally, weapons such as stone-throwing machines were used to get rid of attackers.

___ Castles were also made with very thick walls.

___ They were built at places hard for enemies to reach.

___ In the Middle Ages, people built castles to defend themselves from attack.

---

15. ___ When he woke he had strange psychic powers.

___ He received a concussion from the fall and remained unconscious for three days.

___ These pictures were of people and places that he had never seen.

___ Peter Hurkos was an ordinary house painter until he fell off a ladder.

___ The powers enabled him to see pictures flashing through his mind.

___ These powers have come to be known as "psychometrics."

Target Area 6: Syllogisms

DIRECTIONS: The following sentences have a logical relationship to each other. The conclusions also follow logically. Read exactly what is written down and then write a conclusion based on the information given.

EXAMPLE: All dogs have four legs.

My pet is a dog.

Therefore my pet must have *four legs.*

1. All robins have red breasts.

   This bird is a robin.

   Therefore this bird has ______________________________

2. All balls cost a quarter.

   This is a ball.

   Therefore it costs ______________________________

3. Things made of wood can burn.

   This is made of wood.

   Therefore it ______________________________

4. All birds lay eggs.

   Quails are birds.

   Therefore quails ______________________________

5. Food made with sugar is fattening.

   Cake is made with sugar.

   Therefore cake is ______________________________

6. All humans have fingernails.

   Joe is a human.

   Therefore Joe ______________________________

7. All eighteen-year-olds can vote.

   Sharon is eighteen years old.

   Therefore Sharon ______________________________

8. All fish swim.

   Flounder are fish.

   Therefore flounder ______________________________

9. All bananas have yellow skin.

   This fruit is a banana.

   Therefore it has ______________________________

10. All new cars cost over $4,000.

    This is a new car.

    Therefore this car ______________________________

11. Ralph is a yellow bird.

    All birds fly except yellow birds.

    Can Ralph fly? ______________________________

12. You can buy nails only at a hardware store.

    This is a drugstore.

    Can you buy nails here? ______________________________

13. All ten-year old girls like dolls.

    Joan is a girl.

    Must Joan like dolls? ______________________________

14. Black cows are Holsteins.

Brown cows are Guernseys.

Bessy is an Ayrshire.

Do you know anything else about her? ______________________

15. Harry and Ann went to the beach.

There were many children at the beach.

Do Harry and Ann have to be children? ______________________

16. Liz is older than John.

John is older than Jim.

Who is oldest? ______________________

17. My cup holds less than my glass.

My glass holds more than my mug.

Which holds the most? ______________________

18. Carol is stronger than Jane.

Mary is stronger than Carol.

Is Mary stronger than Jane? ______________________

19. Harry is faster than Lloyd.

Lloyd is slower than Ted.

Ted is ______________________ than Lloyd.

20. Lynn and Nancy are taller than Meg.

Kathy and Nancy are the same height.

Lynn is taller than Kathy.

Who is tallest? ______________________

Who is shortest? ______________________

21. I am smarter than my sister.

    My sister is smarter than my brother.

    My brother is ________________________ than I am.

22. Apples and oranges are larger than cherries and smaller than cantalope.

    Apples are ________________________ than cantalope.

23. Rob is taller than Sam.

    Sam is taller than Bill.

    Sam is shorter than ________________________

24. Honey is sweeter than maple syrup.

    Maple syrup is sweeter than sugar.

    Molasses is less sweet than sugar.

    Maple syrup is ________________________ than sugar.

25. I like carrots better than beans.

    I like beans better than corn.

    I like peas more than carrots.

    What do I like most? ________________________

    What do I like least? ________________________

Target Area 7

USE OF ABSTRACT REASONING

The aphasic patient typically finds abstract reasoning activities much more challenging than concrete reasoning tasks; he is therefore much less confident when approaching questions that demand abstract reasoning skills. Target Area Seven provides exercises that may aid the patient in improving these skills and increase his confidence when he confronts them.

The initial two exercises are rather uncomplicated and allow the patient necessary practice in basic abstract reasoning. The remaining exercises in this section are increasingly difficult. As in other target areas, the responses solicited here range from a single word to a sentence. The exercises with proverbs are the final group in this section: they are the most abstract and demand the greatest number of reasoning skills. Although an aphasic may be able to fit a particular proverb to a given situation, he is often unable to translate the meaning into his own words, in order to give a good example. The exercises with proverbs encourage this activity and, as the questions ask the patient for his feelings and opinions, they may spark valuable discussion. Many of these exercises may also be used successfully in group sessions.

M.R.

Target Area 7: Intangibles

DIRECTIONS: Write the answers to the following questions.

EXAMPLE: Give an example of something cold. *ice*

1. Give an example of something painful.

   ____

2. Give an example of something courageous.

   ____

3. Give an example of something tragic.

   ____

4. Give an example of something fluffy.

   ____

5. Give an example of something soft.

   ____

6. Give an example of something slippery.

   ____

7. Give an example of something inflatable.

   ____

8. Give an example of something that hurts your ears.

   ____

9. Give an example of something sour.

   ____

10. Give an example of something that is an imitation of something else. ____________________

11. Give an example of something opaque.

    ____

12. Give an example of something that fizzes.

    ____

13. Give an example of something smooth.

____

14. Give an example of something shiny.

____

15. Give an example of something that needs tuning.

____

16. Give an example of something that is unpleasant.

____

17. Give an example of something bitter.

____

18. Give an example of something that is loving.

____

19. Give an example of something that melts.

____

20. Give an example of something that has to be renewed.

____

21. Give an example of something stiff.

____

22. Give an example of something pliable.

____

23. Give an example of something that changes shape.

____

24. Give an example of something that should be polished.

____

25. Give an example of something that should be insured.

____

26. Give an example of something illegal.

____

27. Give an example of something that needs to be planned.

____

28. Give an example of something that needs to be repeated.

____

29. Give an example of something comical.

____

30. Give an example of something you wind up.

____

31. Give an example of something that has springs.

____

32. Give an example of something that might expire.

____

33. Give an example of something that tastes sweet.

____

34. Give an example of something that is extinct.

____

35. Give an example of something dangerous.

____

36. Give an example of something fake.

____

37. Give an example of something you enjoy doing.

____

38. Give an example of something habit forming.

____

39. Give an example of something that changes color.

____

40. Give an example of something wider than it is high.

____

Target Area 7: Incongruities

DIRECTIONS: The following sentences do not make logical sense. Rewrite the sentences so that they make sense.

EXAMPLE: I was so cold that I was perspiring.

I was so hot that I was perspiring.

1. I opened my eyes really wide and heard the birds in the trees.

2. I am going to skip lunch because I am really starved.

3. I am the world's smallest giant.

4. I turned the radio on so that I could watch the movie.

5. The first wound killed the victim, the second one only stunned him.

6. Perfume tastes good, but it smells terrible.

7. He took ten pictures after he ran out of film.

8 It was so hot that we turned the thermostat up five degrees.

9. The violinist knew that every instrument was out of tune except his.

10. He was sleeping so soundly that he woke up every three minutes.

11. He was brushing his hair with a new toothbrush.

12. Nobody answered the phone when I called John, so I talked with him for fifteen minutes.

13. The bases were loaded so they attempted a field goal.

14. My brother's wife is my mother-in-law.

15. I became so hot walking through the jungle that I stopped and warmed my feet by the fire.

16. The birds were flying south to Alaska to avoid the cold weather.

17. I finished the main course just as the waitress brought in the appetizer.

18. My deaf brother said he heard some funny jokes on television last night.

19. I saw a man on the radio who was wearing a red plaid coat.

20. The ink in my pencil ran out.

21. When I saw that it was snowing, I put on my sandals.

22. I was so thirsty that I ate some crackers.

23. She unlocked the door so no one could get in.

24. At night I turn off the lights so I can see better.

25. It was such a good television program that I went backstage and congratulated the actors.

26. I shut the book and started reading.

27. I put the casserole in the freezer to heat, and got the ice cream from the oven.

28. The water was so cold that I put on my wool coat before I went swimming.

29. We lit the firecracker on top of his birthday cake.

30. My checks bounced because I had too much money in my account.

31. I needed my flashlight because it was so bright.

32. The giraffe's neck was so long that he could reach only the lowest bushes.

33. There is a new dandelion exhibit at the zoo.

34. The man decided to grow a toupee after his hair fell out.

35. His wife held out her thumb so that her new ring could be fitted.

36. He swore on a stack of comics that he would tell the truth.

37. The cat was so afraid of the mouse that he cowered in the corner with fright.

38. The parking meter needed another crime so that it wouldn't expire.

39. Franklin Delano Rockefeller was a fine President.

40. Teaching me to play tennis is like trying to give an old dog new bones.

Target Area 7: Analogies, Exercise 1

DIRECTIONS: The following are analogies. There is a relationship between the first two words. Write a word in the blank that makes the relationship between the third and fourth words the **same** as that between the first and second words. Choose the correct word from the choices that are given.

EXAMPLE: **Up** is to **down** as **in** is to out

out above enter

1. **Black** is to **white** as **hot** is to ______

color cold warm

2. **Big** is to **small** as **elephant** is to ______

peanuts animal ant

3. **Hand** is to **glove** as **foot** is to ______

feet shoe ankle

4. **Jelly** is to **jar** as **eggs** are to ______

carton hen food

5. **Eye** is to **see** as **ear** is to ______

hear eardrum head

6. **Wing** is to **bird** as **fin** is to ______

fish finish handle

7. **Shoe** is to **foot** as **hat** is to ______

coat head sombrero

8. **Beverage** is to **drink** as **cake** is to ______

chocolate icing eat

9. **Mother** is to **father** as **aunt** is to ______________

uncle relative cousin

---

10. **Student** is to **teacher** as **child** is to ______________

parent doll obey

---

11. **Bird** is to **nest** as **man** is to ______________

city house chirp

---

12. **Winter** is to **summer** as **fall** is to ______________

spring season October

---

13. **Corn** is to **vegetable** as **pineapple** is to ______________

fruit Hawaii apple

---

14. **Chop suey** is to **Chinese** as **spaghetti** is to ______________

German Italian sauce

---

15. **Soldier** is to **army** as **sailor** is to ______________

Wac navy sea

---

16. **Child** is to **younger** as **adult** is to ______________

grownup older person

---

17. **Gasoline** is to **car** as **food** is to ______________

man eat refrigerator

---

18. **Bread** is to **carbohydrate** as **meat** is to ______________

vitamins protein starch

---

19. **Table** is to **wood** as **mirror** is to ______________

cement glass stand

---

20. **Skin** is to **man** as **feathers** are to ______________

birds covering woman

21. **Snow** is to **flake** as **rain** is to ____________________

cloudy weather drop

22. **Mayor** is to **city** as **governor** is to ____________________

country state town

23. **Yarn** is to **knit** as **thread** is to ____________________

needle sew thimble

24. **Keys** are to **piano** as **strings** are to ____________________

drums trumpet violin

25. **East** is to **west** as **north** is to ____________________

direction south southern

26. **Pyramid** is to **triangle** as **cube** is to ____________________

four sides square rectangle

27. **Mother** is to **daughter** as **father** is to ____________________

son grandfather parent

28. **Buy** is to **sell** as **open** is to ____________________

door product close

29. **Day** is to **night** as **sun** is to ____________________

sunlight moon sunset

30. **Seven** is to **eight** as **eleven** is to ____________________

twelve lucky seventeen

31. **August** is to **July** as **May** is to ____________________

November January April

32. **Button** is to **shirt** as **zipper** is to ____________________

fastener track pants

33. **Second** is to **minute** as **minute** is to ______________

time hour day

34. **Above** is to **below** as **top** is to ______________

surface bottom side

35. **Boat** is to **dock** as **car** is to ______________

road automobile garage

36. **Alike** is to **same** as **unlike** is to ______________

opposite different variety

37. **Seam** is to **team** as **sap** is to ______________

tap tree top

38. **Green** is to **grass** as **black** is to ______________

coal grey color

39. **Peninsula** is to **land** as **bay** is to ______________

dock water boats

40. **Notes** are to **music** as **words** are to ______________

speech dictionary screaming

41. **Pink** is to **red** as **beige** is to ______________

brown color green

42. **Knobs** are to **doors** as **keys** are to ______________

keychains wallets locks

43. **Bamboo** is to **wood** as **mango** is to

bananas fruit maple

Target Area 7: Analogies, Exercise 2

DIRECTIONS: Choose a word to fill the blank that will make the relationship correct. The relationship between the third word and the word you choose should be the **same** as that between the first and second words.

EXAMPLE: **Up** is to **down** as **in** is to out

1. **Right** is to **wrong** as **good** is to ______________________
2. **Dime** is to **ten** as **quarter** is to ______________________
3. **Beef** is to **cow** as **pork** is to ______________________
4. **Siamese** is to **cat** as **poodle** is to ______________________
5. **Bat** is to **baseball** as **racket** is to ______________________
6. **Rich** is to **poor** as **fat** is to ______________________
7. **Bee** is to **insect** as **blue jay** is to ______________________
8. **Dinner** is to **eat** as **book** is to ______________________
9. **Cow** is to **moo** as **duck** is to ______________________
10. **Blue** is to **color** as **Chevrolet** is to ______________________
11. **Saturday** is to **day** as **February** is to ______________________
12. **Husband** is to **wife** as **man** is to ______________________
13. **Fingers** are to **hands** as **toes** are to ______________________
14. **Coffee** is to **drink** as **cigarette** is to ______________________
15. **Couch** is to **living room** as **stove** is to ______________________
16. **Rug** is to **floor** as **paintings** are to ______________________
17. **Lansing** is to **Michigan** as **Albany** is to ______________________
18. **Sleep** is to **bed** as **sit** is to ______________________

19. **Ounce** is to **pound** as **pint** is to ________________

20. **Sugar** is to **sweet** as **vinegar** is to ________________

21. **Hard** is to **steel** as **soft** is to ________________

22. **Calf** is to **cow** as **puppy** is to ________________

23. **Green** is to **go** as **red** is to ________________

24. **Sail** is to **boat** as **drive** is to ________________

25. **Electrician** is to **wire** as **carpenter** is to ________________

26. **Fawn** is to **deer** as **chick** is to ________________

27. **Day** is to **week** as **month** is to ________________

28. **Cold** is to **hot** as **winter** is to ________________

29. **Red** is to **cherry** as **yellow** is to ________________

30. **Tape recorder** is to **hear** as **photograph** is to ________________

31. **Goose** is to **geese** as **mouse** is to ________________

32. **Three** is to **number** as **G** is to ________________

33. **Freezer** is to **cold** as **oven** is to ________________

34. **December** is to **January** as **last** is to ________________

35. **Giant** is to **midget** as **huge** is to ________________

36. **Scalpel** is to **surgeon** as **wrench** is to ________________

37. **Pulp** is to **paper** as **hemp** is to ________________

38. **Plum** is to **prune** as **grape** is to ________________

39. **Hamburger** is to **dinner** as **cereal** is to ________________

40. **Group** is to **people** as **herd** is to ________________

Target Area 7: Proverbs, Exercise 1

DIRECTIONS: Each of the following has a phrase in quotes. Pick the one explanation that best interprets what the phrase means. Circle the letter of the correct interpretation.

EXAMPLE: "Actions speak louder than words" most nearly means

a. Actions have a louder voice than anything else.

(b.) What you do is more important than what you say.

c. What you say is more important than what you do.

1. "Every cloud has a silver lining" most nearly means

   a. Clouds are silver in color.

   b. Good can be found in everything.

   c. Everything is worth money.

---

2. "All that glitters is not gold" most nearly means

   a. Something showy isn't always valuable.

   b. Gold glitters, but not everything else does.

   c. Something valuable isn't always expensive.

---

3. "Silence is golden" most nearly means

   a. Money talks.

   b. Pride goes before a fall.

   c. Keeping quiet may be better than saying something.

---

4. "A rolling stone gathers no moss" most nearly means

   a. Constant changes in your life may not lead to success.

   b. Green thumbs are valuable.

   c. Staying active keeps you young.

5. “Jack of all trades” most nearly means
   a. He does business with everyone.
   b. He knows a lot about nothing.
   c. He knows a little about everything.

---

6. “A watched pot never boils” most nearly means
   a. Wishing doesn’t make it come true.
   b. Things happen when you least expect them.
   c. Don’t look for things that won’t come.

---

7. “You can’t have your cake and eat it too” most nearly means
   a. You want everything given to you.
   b. You want food and someone to feed it to you, too.
   c. You expect too much of the world.

---

8. “A little learning is a dangerous thing” most nearly means
   a. Learn what you can, as time is short.
   b. Finding out new things has terrible consequences.
   c. Sometimes knowing only a few facts about something can lead you to misunderstand it.

---

9. “You can’t teach an old dog new tricks” most nearly means
   a. Dogs can’t be taught anything when they are old.
   b. If you are old, it’s harder to learn new things.
   c. You can’t learn unless you’re a dog.

---

10. “Don’t look a gift horse in the mouth” most nearly means
    a. Be thankful for what you have.
    b. Appreciate what you receive.
    c. Don’t accept gifts from horses.

11. "It's like looking for a needle in a haystack" most nearly means
    a. Needles are hard to find in haystacks.
    b. It's better late than never.
    c. It's extremely hard to find.

---

12. "Too many cooks spoil the broth" most nearly means
    a. Two is company, three's a crowd.
    b. It doesn't pay to work too hard.
    c. Having too many people give orders may ruin a project.

---

13. "Don't judge a book by its cover" most nearly means
    a. Watch out for strangers.
    b. Appearances don't always reveal what something is worth.
    c. Books aren't always the same on the inside as they are on the outside.

---

14. "Let sleeping dogs lie" most nearly means
    a. Animals sleep lying down, not standing up.
    b. Dogs have trouble waking up.
    c. Don't stir up an old trouble.

---

15. "The pot calling the kettle black" most nearly means
    a. People who live in glass houses shouldn't throw stones.
    b. Once a sailor, always a sailor.
    c. Haste makes waste.

Target Area 7: Proverbs, Exercise 2

DIRECTIONS: Give an example of how each of the proverbs below has applied to you in real life, or how it could apply to you in a real situation. Write your explanation on another sheet of paper.

EXAMPLE: Actions speak louder than words.

If I tell my friends I'm not afraid of heights, and then go with them to the top of a tall building and start shaking, they will believe I'm afraid of heights in spite of what I'd said.

1. Haste makes waste.
2. Out of sight, out of mind.
3. Don't put all your eggs in one basket.
4. Nothing ventured, nothing gained.
5. Birds of a feather flock together.
6. A stitch in time saves nine.
7. Early to bed and early to rise makes a man healthy, wealthy, and wise.
8. Look before you leap.
9. People who live in glass houses shouldn't throw stones.
10. Mighty oaks from little acorns grow.
11. Don't count your chickens before they're hatched.
12. He who makes no mistakes makes nothing.
13. A penny saved is a penny earned.
14. He's a chip off the old block.
15. In concentration there is strength.

Target Area 7: Proverbs, Exercise 3

DIRECTIONS: On another sheet of paper, explain what each of the proverbs means to you by rewriting it completely. Use your own words.

EXAMPLE: Actions speak louder than words.
What you do means more than what you say.

1. Better late than never.
2. Where there's a will, there's a way.
3. Practice makes perfect.
4. Don't cry over spilled milk.
5. Don't cross your bridges until you come to them.
6. A bird in the hand is worth two in the bush.
7. All work and no play makes Jack a dull boy.
8. Honesty is the best policy.
9. The grass is always greener on the other side of the fence.
10. Take things as they come.
11. An ounce of prevention is worth a pound of cure.
12. Beauty is only skin deep.
13. Don't put off until tomorrow what you can do today.
14. No man is an island unto himself.
15. Blood is thicker than water.

Target Area 8

PERSONAL EXPRESSION

Target Area Eight concentrates on the patient's ability to express complete thoughts in proper written form. Because these questions ask him to record his feelings and opinions carefully, they encourage the aphasic patient to take responsibility for his responses. The exercises in this target area represent the culmination of the aphasia rehabilitation process, the patient's creative use of language. The exercises are designed to aid him in the transition from a reliance on a given structure for his writing to the formulation of his own structures.

All of the exercises may be adapted easily for oral use. The patient's oral answers may well stimulate discussions that will foster more completeness of thought, improved logical inference, and a more orderly sequence of ideas when he later writes his answers. As all of the questions ask for the patient's opinions and feelings, there can be no truly wrong answers; the correctness of his response will lie in his logic, syntax, spelling, and grammar.

M.R.

Target Area 8: Completions

DIRECTIONS: Complete the thought with one or more words. Write them in the blanks provided.

EXAMPLE: I like *flowers* because *they are so colorful and pretty.*

1. I like ______________ because ______________
____

2. I don't like ______________ because ______________
____

3. The trouble with politics is ______________
____

4. You look like ______________
____

5. Snow is ______________
____

6. She came late because ______________
____

7. I wish ______________
____

8. It upsets me to ______________
____

9. Flowers are ______________
____

10. I hope that ______________________________

____

11. Television programs ______________________________

____

12. Why are you ______________________________

____

13. Where is ______________________________

____

14. Mountain climbing is ______________________________

____

15. On rainy days I feel ______________________________

____

16. Newspapers are ______________________________

____

17. I would like to ______________________________

____

18. The President should ______________________________

____

19. It is boring to ______________________________

____

20. My home is ______________________________

____

21. It is against the law to ______________________________
____

22. Why don't you ______________________________
____

23. Clouds are like ______________________________
____

24. Give me the ______________________________
____

25. I want to go ______________________________
____

26. It's very exciting to ______________________________
____

27. I'm looking forward to ______________________________
____

28. Summer ______________________________
____

29. I used to ______________________________
____

30. Money is ______________________________
____

31. You need an invitation to ______________________________
____

32. Frank Sinatra is ______________________________

____

33. There is never enough ______________________________

____

34. I need ______________________________

____

35. I have ______________________________

____

36. If I could, I would ______________________________

____

37. Farmers ______________________________

____

38. Elizabeth Taylor is ______________________________

____

39. The trouble with kids is ______________________________

____

40. It should be a law that ______________________________

____

41. I wonder what it's like to ______________________________

____

42. I'd like to go to ______________________________

____

43. Why ______________________________

____

44. Shopping is ______________________________

____

45. Children are ______________________________

____

46. There is no way that ______________________________

____

47. One of the best ______________________________

____

48. The sale was ______________________________

____

49. Without a doubt ______________________________

____

50. He has a habit of ______________________________

____

51. Because of the weather, ______________________________

____

52. Yesterday ______________________________

____

53. Thirty years ago, ______________________________

____

Target Area 8: Descriptions

DIRECTIONS: In complete sentences write an explanation that answers each question. Be complete and descriptive in your answer. Use another sheet of paper.

EXAMPLE: Describe what a ping pong ball looks like

It's the size of a golf ball and it's used in playing ping pong. It's whit[e,] hollow, lightweight, and bounces well.

1. Describe what you are wearing.
2. Describe the way a banana looks.
3. Describe what emotions are.
4. Describe the room you are in.
5. Describe an object near you.
6. Describe how to get from your home to the closest store.
7. Describe the way a giraffe looks.
8. Describe the way the living room looks where you live.
9. Describe what you do on an average day.
10. Describe how someone you know looks.
11. Describe what you look like.
12. Describe your personality.
13. Describe your strong points.
14. Describe your weaknesses.
15. Describe a fruit without telling its name.
16. Describe a vegetable without telling its name.
17. Describe something you would like to have.
18. Describe a place you have visited.
19. Describe your feelings about smoking.

20. Describe what a friend is.
21. Describe what love is.
22. Describe what a stained glass window is.
23. Describe what you think living on Mars would be like.
24. Describe something beautiful.
25. Describe something ugly.
26. Describe something you enjoy doing.
27. Describe the personality of some member of your family.
28. Describe the qualities a good President should have.
29. Describe a rainbow.
30. Describe what you feel like right now.
31. Describe how you would feel if you had a terminal illness.
32. Describe what zero gravity would be like.
33. Describe your feet in detail.
34. Describe a food item you like.
35. Describe the way a cat washes itself.
36. Describe an article of your clothing.
37. Pick something and describe how it smells.
38. Describe how you would change a part of your home.
39. Describe the man/woman of your dreams.
40. Describe where you would like to spend a vacation.
41. Describe the "one that got away."
42. Describe what you see outside the nearest window.
43. Describe how a computer could help the average person.
44. Describe how to be a good friend.
45. Describe a goal you have for yourself.

Target Area 8: Opinions

DIRECTIONS: Below are questions that ask you for your opinion. On another sheet of paper, write a full answer to each question.

EXAMPLE: If you could have one month last all year long, which month would it be and why?

I would have September last all year, because the temperature is pleasant and the leaves are turning.

1. If you could have three wishes come true, what would they be?
2. If you could meet any living person in the world, whom would you want to meet and why?
3. If you were President, what is the first law you would make?
4. If you were given $500,000 how would you use it?
5. If you were to write a book, what would you write about?
6. If, overnight, you could become an expert on any subject, what subject would you choose, and why?
7. If you had to choose between being either blind or deaf, which one would you choose, and why?
8. If you could take a trip to any place in the world, where would you go, why would you choose to go there, and what would you most want to see?
9. If a fine chef were going to prepare a feast for you, what would you want the menu to include?

10. If you could redesign the automobile, what things would you change, and why?

11. If you had to be an animal, what kind of animal would you be, and why?

12. If you gave a lecture on how to treat someone who has had a stroke, what would you say?

13. If you were able to read another person's mind, would you do it? Why or why not?

14. If someone were to pay for you to live for six months anywhere in the world, where would you choose to live, and why?

15. If you were able to see into your own future, would you want to do it? Why or why not?

16. If you could change one thing in your life, what would it be, and why?

17. If you could have a conversation with a famous person who is now dead, whom would you choose? What questions would you ask him or her?

18. If you were stranded on a desert island and could choose one person to be with you, whom would you choose, and why?

19. If you had food and were going to be alone in a forest for two weeks, what would you do to pass the time?

20. If you were designing your dream house and didn't need to worry about money, what features would it include? What style would it be? What would the rooms be like? How big would it be? Where would it be?

21. If you could change one event in your past, what would it be and how would you change it?

22. If you could excel instantly at any occupation, which one would you choose, and why?

23. If you wrote a newspaper column distributed all over the United States, what would you write about and why would you choose that topic?

24. If you could live during any other period in history, when would you live, and why?

25. If you could solve any problem, what would be the problem you would choose? How would you solve it, and why is it important that it be solved?

26. If you could know when it is you are going to die, would you want to know it? Why or why not?

27. If you could choose to be a certain age forever, what age would you choose, and why?

28. If you could prevent any one person from doing one specific thing, who would you choose and what would you prevent him or her from doing?

29. If you could change one aspect of your personality, what would it be? Why would you change it?
30. If you were to pick the most important thing you've learned during your life, what would it be? Why is it important to you?
31. If you could talk with one of your dead relatives, who would you choose and what would you talk about?
32. If you could live in a different state, where would you live and why?
33. If you were offered private lessons of some type from a famous person, who would you study with and why?
34. If you were going to be a contestant on a quiz show, which one would you pick and why?
35. If you could change some of your physical characteristics, what would you change and why?
36. If you were to become famous, what would you like to be known for and why?
37. If you had named yourself at birth, what names would you have chosen and why?
38. If you could have a date with any famous living person, who would you choose and why?
39. If you could learn to play a musical instrument, which one would you choose and why?
40. If you could own a second home, where would it be and why?

Target Area 8: Hypothetical Situations

DIRECTIONS: On another sheet of paper, answer the following questions with complete sentences.

EXAMPLE: What would you do if your clothes were too small?
I would either buy new clothes or lose some weight.

1. What would you do if the zipper broke on your pants or dress while you were shopping?
2. What would you do if you had lost your wallet?
3. What would you do if you spilled food on your clothes?
4. What would you do if you wanted to find out how a word is spelled?
5. What would you do if the electricity in your home went off?
6. What would you do if you witnessed a robbery?
7. What would you do if a waitress in a restaurant brought you the wrong order?
8. What would you do if you had forgotten an important phone number?
9. What would you do if you had been bitten by a snake?
10. What would you do if you found out that someone you trust had lied to you?

11. What would you do if a package that belonged to someone else was delivered to you?
12. What would you do if you found a $100 dollar bill on the sidewalk?
13. What would you do if you locked yourself out of your home?
14. What would you do if you ran out of gas on an expressway?
15. What would you do if a fire started in your room?
16. What would you do if you needed information about insect bites?
17. What would you do if you fell in a mud puddle on your way to a party?
18. What would you do if you were invited to a banquet at the White House?
19. What would you do if you wanted to know how to make cornbread?
20. What would you do if you were choking on a piece of food?
21. What would you do if you discovered termites had been eating your furniture?
22. What would you do if you forgot a friend's name?
23. What would you do if you lost your charge cards?
24. What would you do if you got lost on your way to an important meeting?
25. What would you do if the brakes failed while you were driving a car?

26. What would you do if your home was flooded?

27. What would you do if a filling fell out of your tooth?

28. What would you do if you by accident left a party with someone else's coat?

29. What would you do if your finger got stuck in a faucet?

30. What would you do if you were eating and found a bug in your salad?

31. What would you do if your luggage was lost when you took a plane trip?

32. What would you do if you had gone to the theater or a sports event but forgotten your ticket?

33. What would you do if your stove started smoking?

34. What would you do if you were leaving to catch a plane and relatives showed up unexpectedly?

35. What would you do if you saw someone faint in a department store?

36. What would you do if a stranger wanted to come into your home to sell you something?

37. What would you do if you dialed the wrong phone number for a long distance call?

38. What would you do if you got stuck in an elevator?

39. What would you do if one of your close friends told you he or she had committed a crime?

40. What would you do if you had the hiccups?

41. What would you do if you were told to report for jury duty?

42. What would you do if a smoke alarm in the kitchen went off when you were cooking?

43. What would you do if you saw someone choking?

44. What would you do if you had a leak in your ceiling?

45. What would you do if you found termites in your home?

46. What would you do if you accidentally took an overdose of your prescribed medicine?

47. What would you do if you wanted to move some heavy furniture?

48. What would you do if you left a store without your package?

49. What would you do if your refrigerator suddenly stopped working?

50. What would you do if a friend insisted on driving even though he or she had been drinking?

SUPPLEMENTARY MATERIALS

This final group of exercises, as the title indicates, supplements the eight preceding target areas. These exercises are not arranged in an ascending order of difficulty. Most are concerned primarily with word recall, but they demand of the patient the use of a number of different language skills. There is also great diversity among the formats used.

Only two of the exercises ask that a full sentence be written; six require the recognition and copying of a one word answer. While all of the exercises employ everyday language, the clinician will find that their structures can easily accommodate more sophisticated language and material.

M.R.

Supplementary Materials, Exercise 1

DIRECTIONS: These are mini-crossword puzzles. Fill in the squares with a letter which will form words going across and down.

EXAMPLE:

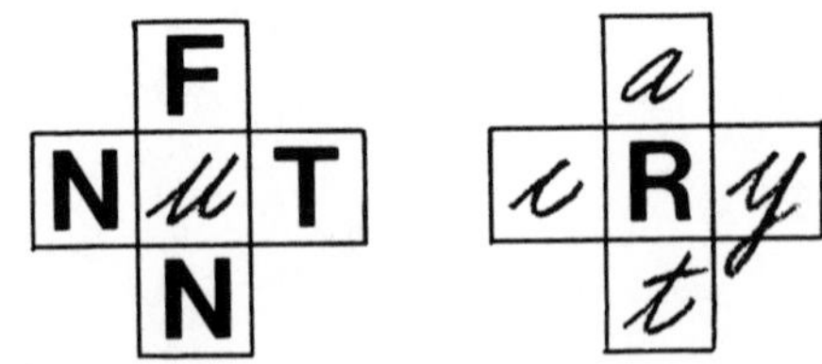

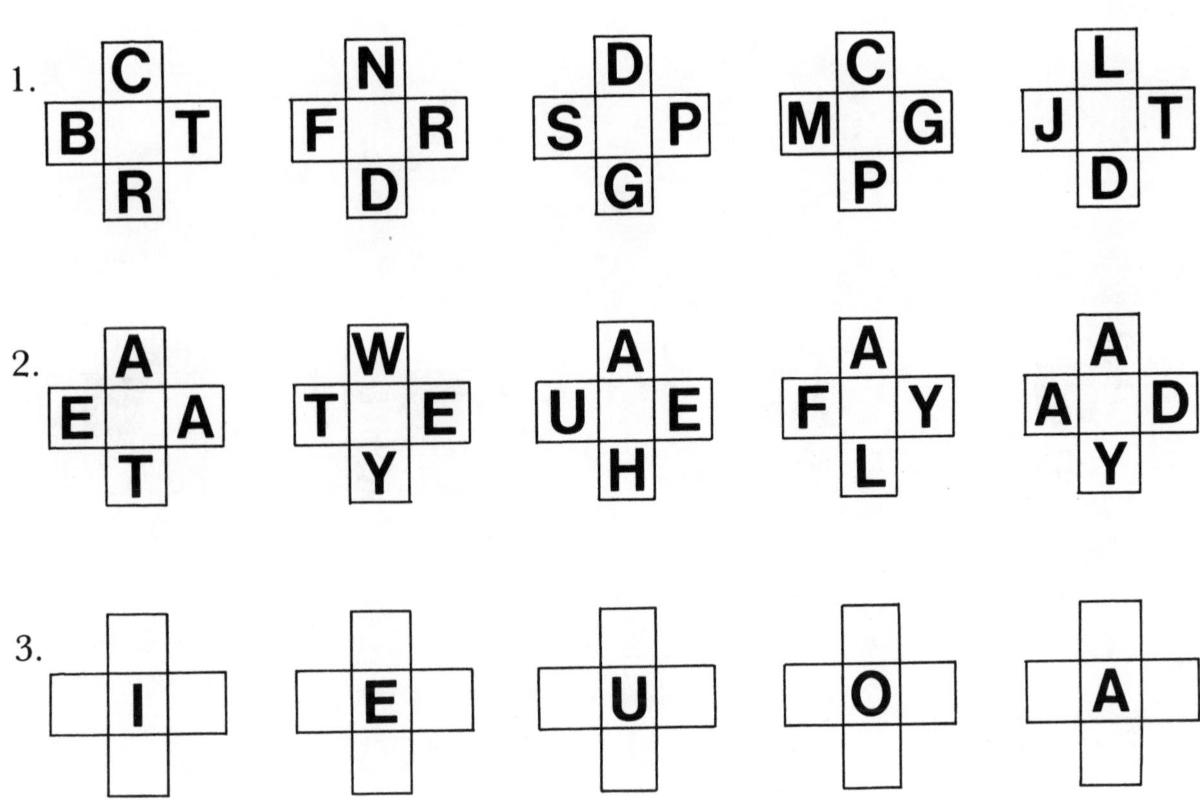

4\.

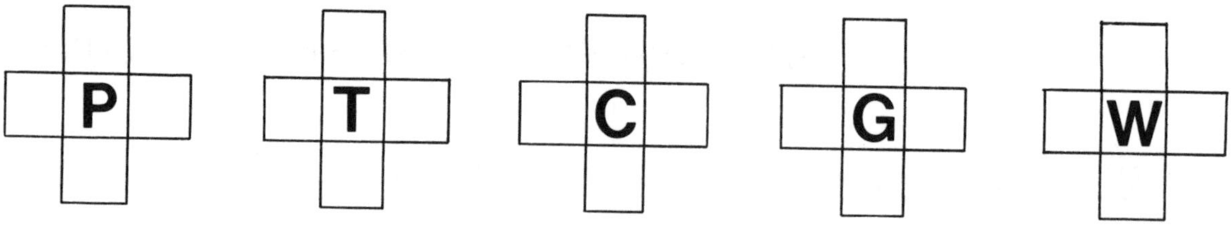

P	T	C	G	W

5\.

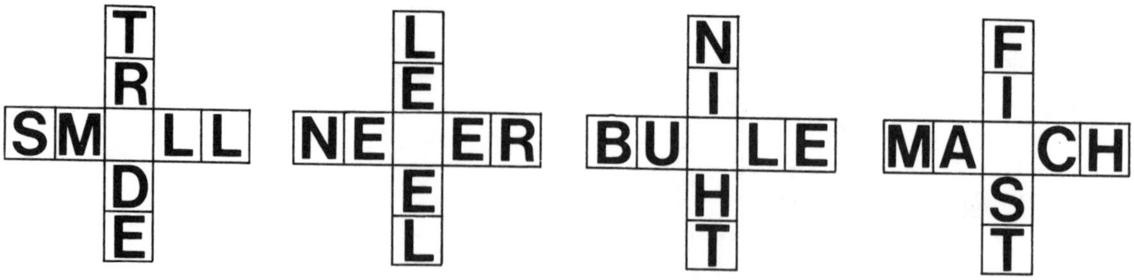

Across	Down
SM _ LL	TR _ DE
NE _ ER	LE _ EL
BU _ LE	NI _ HT
MA _ CH	FI _ ST

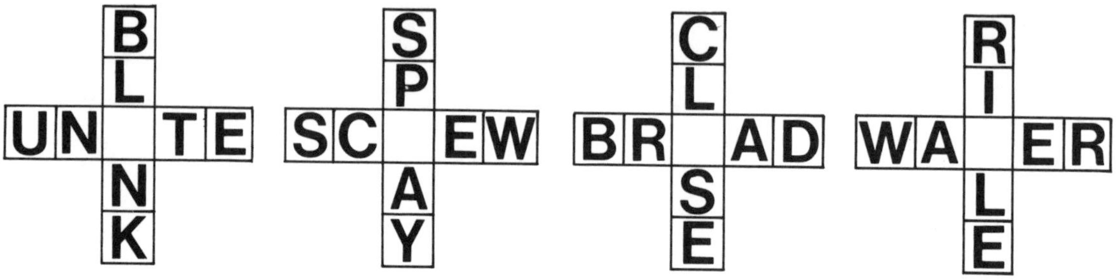

6\.

Across	Down
UN _ TE	BL _ NK
SC _ EW	SP _ AY
BR _ AD	CL _ SE
WA _ ER	RI _ LE

7\.

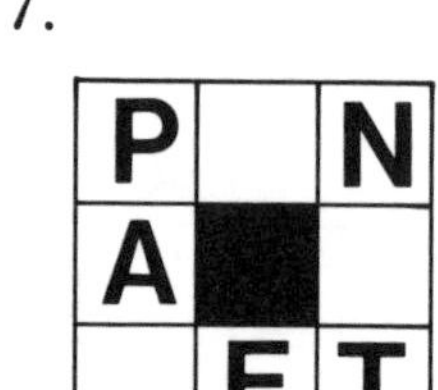

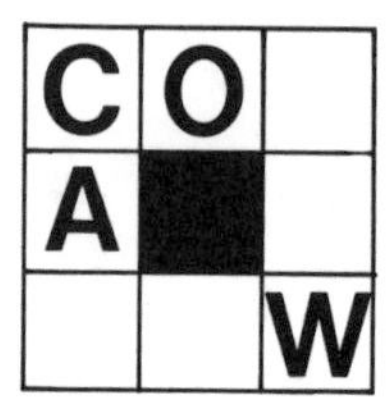

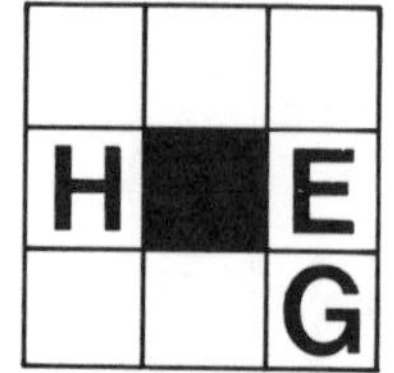

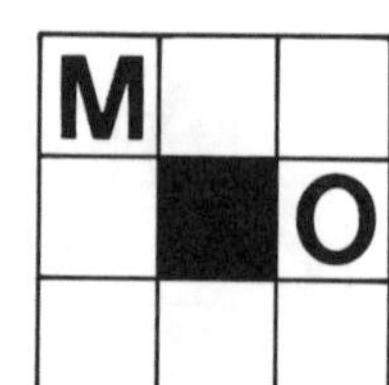

8\.

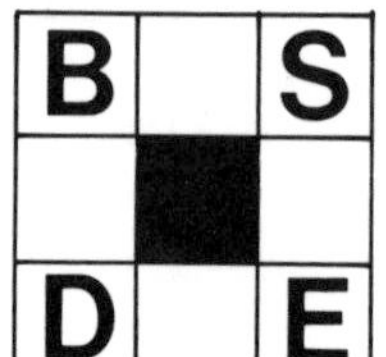

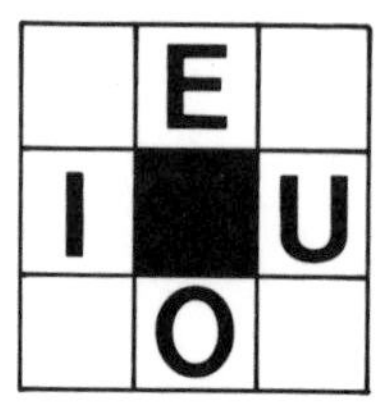

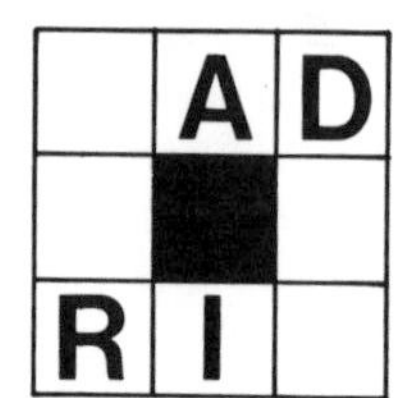

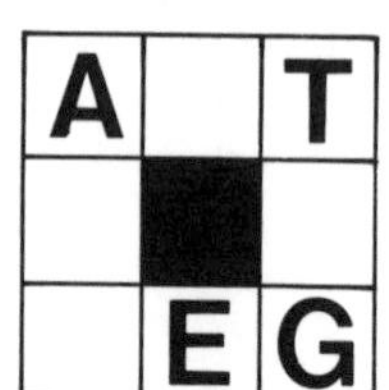

Supplementary Materials, Exercise 2

DIRECTIONS: Below are three columns of syllables. Pick one syllable from each column and put them in the right order, to form a word. The first eight words will be states, the second eight will be cars. The first state is already completed as an example. Hint: Cross out each syllable as you use it.

1. **States**

~~Mich~~	a	ho	Michigan
I	con	ton	______
New	nes	see	______
Wash	Hamp	da	______
Nev	da	shire	______
Wis	~~i~~	~~gan~~	______
Ar	ing	sas	______
Ten	kan	sin	______

2. **Cars**

Chev	il	bile	______
Volks	der	let	______
Pon	wa	ta	______
Olds	cu	bird	______
Mer	ro	gen	______
Cad	ti	lac	______
Toy	o	ry	______
Thun	mo	ac	______

Supplementary Materials, Exercise 3

DIRECTIONS: The following lists of words fall into several categories. Write the letter of the correct category after each word. The first word has been done as an example.

1. Write **d** for desserts, **v** for vegetables, **f** for fruits, or **b** for beverages next to the word.

kumquat *f*	scallions _____	daiquiri _____
artichoke _____	sherry _____	mousse _____
mango _____	sherbet _____	sauerkraut _____
tapioca _____	tangerine _____	cherries jubilee _____
okra _____	eggnog _____	kiwi _____

2. Write **u** if the place is in the United States, **e** if it is in Europe, or **n** if it is not in either one.

Gobi Desert _____	Equator _____	The Vatican _____
Waikiki _____	Taj Mahal _____	Ottawa _____
Vietnam _____	Moscow _____	The Louvre _____
Notre Dame Cathedral _____	Niagara Falls _____	The Alamo _____
Alps _____	Fisherman's Wharf _____	Independence Hall _____
Pentagon _____	Siberia _____	Antarctica _____

Supplementary Materials, Exercise 4

DIRECTIONS: The words at the left are hidden among the letters on the right. The words may be written left to right or top to bottom. When you find the words, circle them. One word has already been done as an example. A letter may be used in more than one word.

Word List 1

angry
bold
brave
confused
coy
excited
glad
joyful
loving
mad
sad
shy
timid

c	a	s	a	n	g	r	y
o	j	o	y	f	u	l	l
n	c	m	n	b	b	u	o
f	o	a	t	o	r	a	v
u	y	d	i	l	a	s	i
s	h	y	m	d	v	a	n
e	x	c	i	t	e	d	g
d	r	p	d	g	l	a	d

DIRECTIONS: The words on the left can be found somewhere among the letters on the right. They may be written top to bottom or bottom to top or left to right. They may be written backwards. An example of a word written backwards is circled and crossed out on the list to give you a start. Locate all of the listed words among the letters on the right, and then circle them. A letter may be used in more than one word.

Word List 2

about
bones
~~bead~~
cares
crazy
graze
juice
later
leads
money
purse
radar
robes
score
sweet
truth
worms

w o l a b o u t
s w e e t a c e
c r a z y n a c
o a d a e b r i
r d s r n o e u
e a e g o n s j
t r b l m e r d
a w o r m s u a
l t r u t h p s

Supplementary Materials, Exercise 5

DIRECTIONS: Each nonsense word below contains two real words. The letters for both words are in the proper order, but they are mixed together. The category gives a hint as to what the two words are. Write them on the line below the nonsense word. The first letter of each word is capitalized.

EXAMPLE: (animals) D C a o t g D *Dog*

C *Cat*

1. These nonsense words each contain two spices or seasonings.

S P e a p p l e t r

S ________________

P ________________

C l S a o v e g e s

C ________________

S ________________

O r e G a g r a l i c n o

O ________________

G ________________

N u t C i n m e n a m g o n

N ________________

C ________________

2. These nonsense words each contain two types of cheeses.

C h e S w d d i a s r s

C ____________________

S ____________________

E d a P a r m m e s a n

E ____________________

P ____________________

A m e F r i e t c a a n

A ____________________

F ____________________

M o z z R o a q u e r f e o l r l t a

M ____________________

R ____________________

---

3. These nonsense words each contain two types of cars.

F D o r d o d g e

F ____________________

D ____________________

C h e P v r o i n l e t t o

C ____________________

P ____________________

L i T o y n o c o t l a n

L ____________________

T ____________________

P o C h r n y t i s a l e r c

P ____________________

C ____________________

Supplementary Materials, Exercise 6

DIRECTIONS: Below are lists of syllables and some definitions. The definitions describe a word. The first syllable of that word is given. Look at the syllables and pick the ones needed to complete the word. Cross out each syllable as you use it. The first word is done as an example. **These are all three-syllable words.**

1. **Syllables:** a lin ~~e~~ mel ber cum o ten ~~phant~~ ant

   a large African animal

   e l e p h a n t

   a chewy type of candy

   c a r ___ ___ ___ ___

   high rank in the Navy

   l i e u ___ ___ ___ ___ ___ ___

   salad vegetable

   c u ___ ___ ___ ___ ___ ___

   stringed instrument

   v i ___ ___ ___ ___

2. **Syllables:** min na ton ue graph ka to as tin do

to keep going

c o n ___ ___ ___ ___ ___

outdoor sport

b a d ___ ___ ___ ___ ___ ___

kind of storm

t o r ___ ___ ___ ___

picture by a camera

p h o ___ ___ ___ ___ ___ ___ ___

a state

A l ___ ___ ___ ___

---

3. **Syllables:** to man gan nut ly a ry lice co ize

put together and arrange

o r ___ ___ ___ ___ ___ ___

what happened in the past

h i s ___ ___ ___ ___

person who makes an arrest

p o ___ ___ ___ ___ ___ ___ ___

a hard fruit

c o ___ ___ ___ ___ ___

a country in Europe

I t ___ ___ ___

Supplementary Materials, Exercise 7

DIRECTIONS: Below are definitions of words and blanks for filling in the words. The number of blanks shows the number of letters missing. Part of the word is given as a clue. The first one is done as an example.

1. The answers all contain the word **run.**

   a. Second place in a competition.

   r u n _n_ _e_ _r_ - _u_ _p_

   b. Average, ordinary stuff

   r u n - ___ ___ - ___ ___ ___ -

   ___ ___ ___ ___

   c. The best hit in baseball ___ ___ ___ ___ r u n

   d. A type of car accident

   ___ ___ ___ ___ ___ ___ r u n

   e. A first testing of something.

   ___ ___ ___ ___ ___ r u n

---

2. The answers all contain the word **jack.**

   a. A toy with a lid that pops off

   j a c k - ___ ___ - ___ ___ ___ - ___ ___ ___

   b. Someone who is handy in many areas

   j a c k ___ ___ ___ ___ ___

   ___ ___ ___ ___ ___ ___

   c. A pumpkin with a face

   j a c k - ___ - ___ ___ ___ ___ ___ ___ ___

   d. A small cutting utensil j a c k ___ ___ ___ ___ ___

   e. A fictional character who brings cold weather

   J a c k ___ ___ ___ ___ ___

3. The answers all contain the word **blue**

   a. A type of bird b l u e ___ ___ ___

   b. A first prize award

      b l u e ___ ___ ___ ___ ___ ___

   c. A nursery rhyme character who had a horn

      ___ ___ ___ ___ ___ ___ ___ ___ ___ Blue

   d. A type of fruit b l u e ___ ___ ___ ___ ___

   e. Architectural plan b l u e ___ ___ ___ ___ ___

---

4. The answers all contain the word **can.**

   a. Artists paint on this c a n ___ ___ ___

   b. The country north of the U. S. C a n ___ ___ ___

   c. A type of waterway for boats c a n ___ ___

   d. A yellow songbird c a n ___ ___ ___

   e. A politician who is running for office

      c a n ___ ___ ___ ___ ___ ___

---

5. The answers all contain the word **ink.**

   a. A color ___ i n k

   b. An automatic eye movement ___ ___ i n k

   c. To use your mental abilities ___ ___ i n k

   d. A place to wash dishes ___ i n k

   e. Something that waters the lawn

      ___ ___ ___ i n k ___ ___ ___

6. The answers all contain the word **men.**

   a. You order from this in a restaurant m e n __

   b. This is said at the end of a prayer __ m e n

   c. The opposite of men __ __ m e n

   d. A substance used to make sidewalks __ __ m e n __

   e. Another word for graduation

   __ __ __ m e n __ __ m e n __

---

7. The answers all contain the word **the.**

   a. rain, snow, storms __ __ __ t h e __

   b. a place to see movies t h e __ __ __ __

   c. opposite of southern __ __ __ t h e __ __

   d. they keep birds warm __ __ __ t h e __ __

   e. not here t h e __ __

---

8. The answers all contain the word **rag.**

   a. place for cars __ __ r a g __

   b. very brave __ __ __ r a g __ __ __ __

   c. violent anger r a g __

   d. a plant many people are allergic to

   r a g __ __ __ __

   e. try to get someone to do something

   __ __ __ __ __ r a g __

Supplementary Materials, Exercise 8

DIRECTIONS: You are shown a definition of a word. The blanks below it show the correct number of letters in the word. Fill in the blanks with the correct letters. If you put your first two answers together, they make the third answer. So, if you know the first two answers, you will automatically know the third one. If you know the third answer, you can fill in the first two.

EXAMPLE:

a. Short word for automobile

c a r

b. Another word for country

n a t i o n

c. A flower

c a r n a t i o n

1. a. What you put a sock on

___ ___ ___ ___

b. A round toy that bounces

___ ___ ___ ___

c. A sport with touchdowns

___ ___ ___ ___ ___ ___ ___ ___

---

2. a. A short word for automobile

___ ___ ___

b. Decay or spoil

___ ___ ___

c. A vegetable rabbits like

___ ___ ___ ___ ___ ___

3. a. Another word for taxi

___ ___ ___

b. The opposite of out

___ ___

c. A small house made of logs

___ ___ ___ ___ ___

---

4. a. What you hear with

___ ___ ___

b. What you wear on your finger

___ ___ ___ ___

c. A piece of jewelry for a woman

___ ___ ___ ___ ___ ___ ___

---

5. a. The opposite of she

___ ___

b. A nickname of Arthur

___ ___ ___

c. A vital part of the body

___ ___ ___ ___ ___

---

6. a. The opposite of out

___ ___

b. The opposite of go

___ ___ ___ ___

c. Money you earn

___ ___ ___ ___ ___ ___

7. a. The opposite of Ma

   ___ ___

   b. What you pay when you lease something

   ___ ___ ___ ___

   c. An adult who has a child

   ___ ___ ___ ___ ___ ___

---

8. a. What you drive

   ___ ___ ___

   b. What a dog is to a person

   ___ ___ ___

   c. Another word for rug

   ___ ___ ___ ___ ___ ___

---

9. a. Very overweight

   ___ ___ ___

   b. The opposite of him

   ___ ___ ___

   c. Mother's mate

   ___ ___ ___ ___ ___ ___

---

10. a. You put things in this

    ___ ___ ___ ___ ___ ___

    b. Something you read

    ___ ___ ___ ___

    c. Another word for purse

    ___ ___ ___ ___ ___ ___ ___ ___ ___ ___

11. a. You and I

___ ___

b. Being someplace

___ ___

c. Opposite of him

___ ___ ___

d. Rain, snow, sun, etc.

___ ___ ___ ___ ___ ___ ___

---

12. a. A writing utensil with ink

___ ___ ___

b. A game for children

___ ___ ___

c. The opposite of off

___ ___

d. Five-sided building in Washington, D.C.

___ ___ ___ ___ ___ ___ ___ ___

---

13. a. A type of fastener

___ ___ ___ ___

b. To pull behind you

___ ___ ___ ___

c. The opposite of off

___ ___

d. A kind of flower

___ ___ ___ ___ ___ ___ ___ ___ ___ ___

14. a. To pull behind you

___ ___ ___ ___

b. The opposite of off

___ ___

c. To go by plane

___ ___ ___

d. A large insect

___ ___ ___ ___ ___ ___ ___ ___ ___

---

15. a. The opposite of out

___ ___

b. The opposite of yes

___ ___

c. A penny

___ ___ ___ ___

d. Not guilty

___ ___ ___ ___ ___ ___ ___ ___

---

16. a. What shoppers look forward to in August

___ ___ ___ ___ ___

b. according to

___ ___ ___

c. parents' boy

___ ___ ___

d. clerk in a store

___ ___ ___ ___ ___ ___ ___ ___ ___ ___ ___

Supplementary Materials, Exercise 9

DIRECTIONS: There are two definitions given for each of the words below. The definitions are different, but they both define the same word. Figure out what the common word is and write it in the blank next to the definitions.

EXAMPLE: a. To mix or beat very fast

b. Something used on a horse to make him go faster

whip

1. a. What a dog does when he breathes very fast

   b. The bottom half of a suit __________

2. a. A dish to put soup in

   b. A sport that you play in an alley __________

3. a. The opposite of hot

   b. A mild infection __________

4. a. A position on a football team

   b. Fishing gear __________

5. a. What a dog wags

   b. Follow very closely behind __________

6. a. The paper protection around a book

   b. A lightweight piece of clothing __________

7. a. A mammal that lives in cold water

   b. To close very tightly and securely

   c. An official insignia __________

8. a. The center of a peach
   b. A deep hole __________________

9. a. The person who throws baseballs
   b. A container for liquids __________________

10. a. A type of mark
    b. Written form of money __________________

11. a. A variety of something
    b. Sweet and gentle __________________

12. a. A heavy metal
    b. Guide or head something __________________

13. a. A miniature of something
    b. Someone who shows clothes __________________

14. a. A cushion
    b. A stack of paper __________________

15. a. One fourth of something
    b. 25 cents __________________

16. a. To drive one's car ahead of another car
    b. To hand over to another person
    c. A free ticket for an event __________________

Supplementary Materials, Exercise 10

DIRECTIONS: The clues below will help form a word. Figure out what each letter will be from the clue and write it on the line. Put the letters together and write the word that is formed.

EXAMPLE: The 1st letter is in **door** but not in **floor.** d

The 2nd letter is in **hot** but not in **hit.** o

The word is do.

1. The first letter is in **dot** but not in **rot.** ____

   The second letter is in **cream** but not in **cram.** ____

   The third letter is in **little** but not in **tie.** ____

   The fourth letter is in **pitch** but not in **patch.** ____

   The fifth letter is in **never** but not in **newer.** ____

   The sixth letter is in **reach** but not in **charm.** ____

   The seventh letter is in **tear** but not in **mate.** ____

   The word is ________________.

2. The first letter is in **broad** but not in **road.** _____

The second letter is in **angel** but not in **gland.** _____

The third letter is in **extra** but not in **extreme.** _____

The fourth letter is in **shutter** but not in **threshes.** _____

The fifth letter is in **elect** but not in **clear.** _____

The sixth letter is in **single** but not in **snuggle.** _____

The seventh letter is in **fluffy** but not in **lovely.** _____

The eighth letter is in **understand** but not in **stranded.** _____

The ninth letter is in **joyful** but not in **joyous.** _____

The word is ____________________ .

---

3. The first letter is in **date** but not in **debt.** _____

The second letter is in **crown** but not in **crow.** _____

The third letter is in **down** but not in **wind.** _____

The fourth letter is in **born** but not in **robe.** _____

The fifth letter is in **alley** but not in **mellow.** _____

The sixth letter is in **name** but not in **earn.** _____

The seventh letter is in **open** but not in **pencil.** _____

The eighth letter is in **bubble** but not in **rabble.** _____

The ninth letter is in **super** but not in **proud.** _____

The word is ____________________ .

Supplementary Materials, Exercise 11

DIRECTIONS: Fill in the blanks with letters to form the missing word. The first word is done as an example. Each blank stands for one letter.

a. **Famous couples**

1. Antony and C l e o p a t r a
2. Romeo and __ __ __ __ __ __
3. Hansel and __ __ __ __ __ __
4. Laurel and __ __ __ __ __
5. Punch and __ __ __ __
6. Adam and __ __ __
7. Gilbert and __ __ __ __ __ __ __ __
8. Rodgers and

   __ __ __ __ __ __ __ __ __ __ __
9. Lone Ranger and __ __ __ __ __
10. Huntley and

    __ __ __ __ __ __ __ __
11. George Burns and Gracie __ __ __ __ __
12. Kermit the Frog and Miss __ __ __ __ __
13. Edgar Bergen and Charlie

    __ __ __ __ __ __ __ __
14. Steve Lawrence and Eydie __ __ __ __ __
15. Prince Charles and Lady __ __ __ __ __

b. **Famous threesomes**

1. faith, hope, and ___ ___ ___ ___ ___ ___ ___
2. hook, line, and ___ ___ ___ ___ ___ ___
3. tall, dark, and ___ ___ ___ ___ ___ ___ ___ ___
4. Tom, Dick, and ___ ___ ___ ___ ___
5. sugar n' spice n'

   ___ ___ ___ ___ ___ ___ ___ ___ ___ ___

   ___ ___ ___ ___
6. Winken, Blinken, and ___ ___ ___
7. reading, writing, and

   ___ ___ ___ ___ ___ ___ ___ ___ ___ ___
8. eat, drink, and ___ ___   ___ ___ ___ ___ ___
9. Department of Health, Education, and

   ___ ___ ___ ___ ___ ___ ___
10. life, liberty, and the pursuit of

    ___ ___ ___ ___ ___ ___ ___ ___ ___
11. bacon, lettuce, and ___ ___ ___ ___ ___ ___
12. red, white, and ___ ___ ___ ___
13. healthy, wealthy, and ___ ___ ___ ___
14. animal, vegetable, or ___ ___ ___ ___ ___ ___ ___
15. snap, crackle, and ___ ___ ___

c. **Famous middle names**

1. Louisa ___ ___ ___ Alcott
2. Lyndon ___ ___ ___ ___ ___ ___ Johnson
3. Edgar ___ ___ ___ ___ ___ Poe
4. Martin ___ ___ ___ ___ ___ ___ King
5. Billy ___ ___ ___ ___ King
6. John ___ ___ ___ ___ ___ ___ ___ ___ ___ ___ Kennedy
7. Clare ___ ___ ___ ___ ___ Luce
8. John ___ ___ ___ ___ ___ ___ Adams
9. Franklin ___ ___ ___ ___ ___ ___ Roosevelt
10. George ___ ___ ___ ___ ___ ___ ___ ___ ___ ___ Carver

---

d. **Famous first names**

1. ___ ___ ___ ___ ___ ___ ___ ___ ___ ___ ___ Columbus
2. ___ ___ ___ ___ ___ Kissinger
3. ___ ___ ___ ___ ___ Sinatra
4. ___ ___ ___ Vanderbilt
5. ___ ___ ___ ___ ___ ___ Eisenhower
6. ___ ___ ___ ___ Disney
7. ___ ___ ___ ___ ___ ___ ___ Shakespeare
8. ___ ___ ___ ___ ___ ___ ___ Churchill
9. ___ ___ ___ ___ ___ ___ ___ Freud
10. ___ ___ ___ ___ ___ Antoinette

Supplementary Materials, Exercise 12

DIRECTIONS: Fill in the blank with the missing word. Each blank stands for one word. The first one has been done as an example.

a. **Incomplete titles**

1. The Wizard of ___Oz___
2. Around the World in ________ ________
3. Speaker of the ________
4. Who's Afraid of ________ ________
5. The Yellow Rose of ________
6. Jingle ________
7. ________ of Arc
8. ________ the Red-Nosed Reindeer
9. The ________ ________ of America
10. Secretary of ________
11. The ________ Show
12. Webster's ________
13. As the ________ Turns
14. Fiddler on the ________
15. ________ Revenue Service
16. ________ of Liberty
17. ________ with the Wind
18. The Leaning ________ of Pisa
19. Mutiny on the ________
20. New Year's ________

b. **Incomplete quotations**

1. One if by land, ______________ ______________
______________ ______________.

2. Friends, Romans, countrymen, ______________
______________ ______________
______________.

3. Give me liberty or ______________
______________ ______________.

4. Ask not what your country can do for you, ask what you
______________ ______________
______________ ______________
______________.

5. To be or not to be, ______________
____
______________ ______________.

6. One small step for man, one giant ______________
______________ ______________.

7. I came, I saw, ______________ ______________.

8. Children should be seen and ______________
______________.

9. To the victors belong ______________
______________.

10. Never put off until tomorrow what ______________
______________ ______________
______________.

Supplementary Materials, Exercise 13

DIRECTIONS: Some words have more than one meaning, even though they have only one spelling. Write a sentence that uses the word in the way described by the definition.

EXAMPLE: Write a sentence with the word **fine** meaning everything's okay.

It is fine with me if you want to play now.

Write a sentence with the word **fine** meaning a sum of money.

He paid a five dollar library fine yesterday

1. a. Write a sentence with the word **record** meaning what you play on a stereo. ____________________

   ____

   b. Write a sentence with **record** meaning an account of something that happened. ____________________

   ____

2. a. Write a sentence with the word **short** meaning not tall.

   ____

   ____

   b. Write a sentence with **short** meaning an electrical problem.

   ____

   ____

3. a. Write a sentence with the word **dice** meaning cubes with numbers on them. ______________________________

____

b. Write a sentence with **dice** meaning to cut into pieces.

____

____

4. a. Write a sentence with the word **jam** meaning what is put on bread. ______________________________

____

b. Write a sentence with **jam** meaning push or crush in a crowd.

____

____

5. a. Write a sentence with the word **pro** meaning in favor of.

____

____

b. Write a sentence with **pro** meaning professional.

____

____

6. a. Write a sentence with the word **walk** meaning to move by foot.

____

____

b. Write a sentence with **walk** meaning a pathway.

____

____

7. a. Write a sentence with the word **bar** meaning a pole or rod.

____

____

b. Write a sentence with **bar** meaning a place to drink.

____

____

8. a. Write a sentence with the word **ear** meaning the part of a corn plant. ____

____

b. Write a sentence with **ear** meaning what you hear with.

____

____

9. a. Write a sentence with the word **rose** meaning stood up.

____

____

b. Write a sentence with **rose** meaning the flower.

____

____

10. a. Write a sentence with the word **felt** meaning touched.

____

____

b. Write a sentence with **felt** meaning the material.

____

____

Supplementary Materials, Exercise 14

DIRECTIONS: Each of the words below has more than one meaning. Write down two **different** meanings for each word.

EXAMPLE: fine— *good quality, nice*
fine— *money paid as a penalty*

1. tie— ____________________
   tie— ____________________

2. can— ____________________
   can— ____________________

3. pool— ____________________
   pool— ____________________

4. date— ____________________
   date— ____________________

5. change— ____________________
   change— ____________________

6. honey— ____________________
   honey— ____________________

7. yard— ____________________
   yard— ____________________

8. orange— ______________________________

orange— ______________________________

9. bark— ______________________________

bark— ______________________________

10. pupil— ______________________________

pupil— ______________________________

11. ball— ______________________________

ball— ______________________________

12. row— ______________________________

row— ______________________________

13. steer— ______________________________

steer— ______________________________

14. safe— ______________________________

safe— ______________________________

15. pop— ______________________________

pop— ______________________________

Supplementary Materials, Exercise 15

DIRECTIONS: The following are sentences in code. To figure out the code, look at the **chart** above the sentences. Each number corresponds to a letter. Look for the number on the top line of the chart. Look directly below that to find out what letter it stands for. Write that letter on the blank. Continue until you can read the whole sentence. It should be complete and make sense when it is filled out correctly. The first word is done as an example.

chart

numbers	9	15	4	19	25	7	14	2	18	12	24	1	8
letters	a	b	c	d	e	f	g	h	i	j	k	l	m

numbers	3	16	21	10	17	11	5	23	26	13	20	22	6
letters	n	o	p	q	r	s	t	u	v	w	x	y	z

1. g i v e   ___ ___
14 18 26 25   8 25

___ ___ ___ ___ ___ ___ ___   ___ ___
1 18 15 25 17 5 22   16 17

___ ___ ___ ___   ___ ___   ___ ___ ___ ___ ___
14 18 26 25   8 25   19 25 9 5 2

chart

numbers	9	15	4	19	25	7	14	2	18	12	24	1	8
letters	a	b	c	d	e	f	g	h	i	j	k	l	m

numbers	3	16	21	10	17	11	5	23	26	13	20	22	6
letters	n	o	p	q	r	s	t	u	v	w	x	y	z

2\. 9 1 1   14 16 16 19   8 25 3

11 2 16 23 1 19   4 16 8 25

5 16   5 2 25   9 18 19

16 7   5 2 25 18 17

4 16 23 3 5 17 22

3\. 13 18 1 1   8 9 3   25 26 25 17

15 25   17 25 21 1 9 4 25 19

15 22   9   4 16 8 21 23 5 25 17?

chart

numbers	9	15	4	19	25	7	14	2	18	12	24	1	8
letters	a	b	c	d	e	f	g	h	i	j	k	l	m

numbers	3	16	21	10	17	11	5	23	26	13	20	22	6
letters	n	o	p	q	r	s	t	u	v	w	x	y	z

4. ___ ___ ___ ___ ___ ___ ___ ___ ___   ___ ___
9 23 11 5 17 9 1 18 9   18 11

___ ___ ___   ___ ___ ___ ___ ___ ___ ___ ___
5 2 25   11 8 9 1 1 25 11 5

___ ___ ___ ___ ___ ___ ___ ___ ___   ___ ___ ___
4 16 3 5 18 3 25 3 5   9 3 19

___ ___ ___   ___ ___ ___ ___ ___ ___ ___
5 2 25   1 9 17 14 25 11 5

___ ___ ___ ___ ___ ___   ___ ___   ___ ___ ___
18 11 1 9 3 19   18 3   5 2 25

___ ___ ___ ___ ___ .
13 16 17 1 19

chart

numbers	9	15	4	19	25	7	14	2	18	12	24	1	8
letters	a	b	c	d	e	f	g	h	i	j	k	l	m

numbers	3	16	21	10	17	11	5	23	26	13	20	22	6
letters	n	o	p	q	r	s	t	u	v	w	x	y	z

5. ___ ___ ___ ___ ___ ___   ___ ___ ___ ___ ___
9 1 13 9 22 11   4 2 25 4 24

___ ___   ___ ___ ___   ___ ___ ___ ___
5 16   11 25 25   5 2 9 5

___ ___ ___ ___ ___ ___ ___ ___ ___ ___
25 1 25 4 5 17 18 4 9 1

___ ___ ___ ___ ___ ___ ___ ___ ___ ___
9 21 21 1 18 9 3 4 25 11

___ ___ ___   ___ ___ ___ ___ ___ ___
9 17 25   5 23 17 3 25 19

___ ___ ___   ___ ___ ___ ___ ___ ___
16 7 7   15 25 7 16 17 25

___ ___ ___ ___ ___ ___ ___   ___ ___ ___
1 25 9 26 18 3 14   5 2 25

___ ___ ___ ___ ___ .
2 16 23 11 25

DIRECTIONS: Do the following exercises in the same way you did the first five. The letters **in code** are on the top line of the chart. They are not in order. Look directly **below** the code letter for the letter that belongs in the sentence. Put that letter on the blank to form the words. The first four letters are done as an example.

chart

code	O	Y	H	M	C	Z	X	B	S	F	N	A	V
letters	a	b	c	d	e	f	g	h	i	j	k	l	m

code	D	Q	E	K	J	W	R	G	U	I	L	P	T
letters	n	o	p	q	r	s	t	u	v	w	x	y	z

1. *a*　*t* *h* *i* ___ ___　___ ___

O　R B S D X　Q Z

___ ___ ___ ___ ___ ___　___ ___　___

Y C O G R P　S W　O

___ ___ ___　___ ___ ___ ___ ___ ___ ___

F Q P　Z Q J C U C J

---

2. ___ ___ ___ ___ ___ ___ ___　___ ___

D Q R B S D X　S W

___ ___ ___ ___ ___ ___ ___　___ ___ ___

H C J R O S D　Y G R

___ ___ ___ ___ ___　___ ___ ___

M C O R B　O D M

___ ___ ___ ___ ___ .

R O L C W

chart

code	O	Y	H	M	C	Z	X	B	S	F	N	A	V
letters	a	b	c	d	e	f	g	h	i	j	k	l	m

code	D	Q	E	K	J	W	R	G	U	I	L	P	T
letters	n	o	p	q	r	s	t	u	v	w	x	y	z

3. __ __ __ __ __ __ __ __ __ __ __
S V V C M S O R C A P

__ __ __ __ __   __   __ __ __ __
H Q U C J   O   Y G J D

__ __ __ __   __ __ __ __
I S R B   H Q A M

__ __ __ __ __   __ __
I O R C J   R Q

__ __ __ __   __ __ __ __
B C A E   W R Q E

__ __ __   __ __ __ __ .
R B C   E O S D

chart

code	O	Y	H	M	C	Z	X	B	S	F	N	A	V
letters	a	b	c	d	e	f	g	h	i	j	k	l	m

code	D	Q	E	K	J	W	R	G	U	I	L	P	T
letters	n	o	p	q	r	s	t	u	v	w	x	y	z

4. ___ ___ ___ ___ ___   ___ ___ ___ ___ ___
O D X C A   Z O A A W

S D   U C D C T G C A O

S W   R I C D R P

R S V C W   B S X B C J

R B O D   D S O X O J O

Z O A A W .

chart

code	O	Y	H	M	C	Z	X	B	S	F	N	A	V
letters	a	b	c	d	e	f	g	h	i	j	k	l	m

code	D	Q	E	K	J	W	R	G	U	I	L	P	T
letters	n	o	p	q	r	s	t	u	v	w	x	y	z

5. S R   S W   R J G C

R B O R   O   J S D X

O J Q G D M   R B C

V Q Q D   G W G O A A P

S D M S H O R C W

R B O R   J O S D   Q J

W D Q I   S W

H Q V S D X .

Susan Howell Brubaker is Assistant Director of the Speech and Language Pathology Department at William Beaumont Hospital, Royal Oak, Michigan. She has had extensive experience with adults who have suffered communicative loss as a result of neurological dysfunction. She holds the B.S. from St. Lawrence University, Canton, N.Y., the M.S. from Ithaca College, Ithaca, N.Y., and the Certificate of Clinical Competence from the American Speech and Hearing Association.

The book was designed by Elizabeth Hanson. The typeface for the text is Baskerville, based on an original design by John Baskerville in the eighteenth century, and the display is Univers, designed by Adrian Frutiger about 1957. The book is printed on 60 lb. and bound in GBC .035 gauge polyethylene Gebex covers and surelox plastic combs.

Manufactured in the United States of America.

TITLES IN THE WILLIAM BEAUMONT HOSPITAL SPEECH AND LANGUAGE PATHOLOGY SERIES

by Susan Howell Brubaker

Basic Level Workbook for Aphasia

Workbook for Aphasia, revised edition

Workbook for Language Skills

Workbook for Reasoning Skills

Workbook for Cognitive Skills

Sourcebook for Speech, Language and Cognition, BOOK 1

Sourcebook for Speech, Language and Cognotion, BOOK 2

Sourcebook for Speech, Language and Cognition, BOOK 3